TREATMENT OF SOFT TISSUE SARCOMAS

Cancer Treatment and Research

WILLIAM L. MCGUIRE, *series editor*

Livingston R.B. (ed): Lung Cancer 1. 1981. ISBN 90-247-2394-9.
Humphrey G.B., Dehner L.P., Grindey G.B., Acton R.T. (eds): Pediatric Oncology 1. 1981.
ISBN 90-247-2408-2.
DeCosse J.J., Sherlock P. (eds): Gastrointestinal Cancer 1. 1981. ISBN 90-247-2461-9.
Bennett J.M. (ed): Lymphomas 1, including Hodgkin's Disease. 1981. ISBN 90-247-2479-1.
Bloomfield C.D. (ed): Adult Leukemias 1. 1982. ISBN 90-247-2478-3.
Paulson D.F. (ed): Genitourinary Cancer 1. 1982. ISBN 90-247-2480-5.
Muggia F.M. (ed): Cancer Chemotherapy 1. ISBN 90-247-2713-8.
Humphrey G.B., Grindey G.B. (eds): Pancreatic Tumors in Children. 1982. ISBN 90-247-2702-2.
Costanzl J.J. (ed): Malignant Melanoma 1. 1983. ISBN 90-247-2706-5.
Griffiths C.T., Fuller A.F. (eds): Gynecologic Oncology. 1983. ISBN 0-89838-555-5.
Greco A.F. (ed): Biology and Management of Lung Cancer. 1983. ISBN 0-89838-554-7.
Walker M.D. (ed): Oncology of the Nervous System. 1983. ISBN 0-89838-567-9.
Higby D.J. (ed): Supportive Care in Cancer Therapy. 1983. ISBN 0-89838-569-5.
Herberman R.B. (ed): Basic and Clinical Tumor Immunology. 1983. ISBN 0-89838-579-2.
Baker L.H. (ed): Soft Tissue Sarcomas. 1983. ISBN 0-89838-584-9.
Bennett J.M. (ed): Controversies in the Management of Lymphomas. 1983. ISBN 0-89838-586-5.
Humphrey G.B., Grindey G.B. (eds): Adrenal and Endocrine Tumors in Children. 1983. ISBN 0-89838-590-3.
DeCosse J.J., Sherlock P. (eds): Clinical Management of Gastrointestinal Cancer. 1983. ISBN 0-89838-601-2.
Catalona W.J., Ratliff T.L. (eds): Urologic Oncology. 1983. ISBN 0-89838-628-4.
Santen R.J., Manni A. (eds): Diagnosis and Management of Endocrine-related Tumors. 1984.
ISBN 0-89838-636-5.
Costanzi J.J. (ed): Clinical Management of Malignant Melanoma. 1984. ISBN 0-89838-656-X.
Wolf G.T. (ed): Head and Neck Oncology. 1984. ISBN 0-89838-657-8.
Alberts D.S., Surwit E.A. (eds): Ovarian Cancer. 1985. ISBN 0-89838-676-4.
Muggia F.M. (ed): Experimental and Clinical Progress in Cancer Chemotherapy. 1985. ISBN 0-89838-679-9.
Higby D.J. (ed): The Cancer Patient and Supportive Care. 1985. ISBN 0-89838-690-X.
Bloomfield C.D. (ed): Chronic and Acute Leukemias in Adults. 1985. ISBN 0-89838-702-7.
Herberman R.B. (ed): Cancer Immunology: Innovative Approaches to Therapy. 1986. ISBN 0-89838-757-4.
Hansen H.H. (ed): Lung Cancer: Basic and Clinical Aspects. 1986. ISBN 0-89838-763-9.
Pinedo H.M., Verweij J. (eds): Clinical Management of Soft Tissue Sarcomas. 1986. ISBN 0-89838-808-2.
Higby D.J. (ed): Issues in Supportive Care of Cancer Patients. 1986. ISBN 0-89838-816-3.
Surwit E.A., Alberts D.S. (eds): Cervix Cancer. 1987. ISBN 0-89838-822-8.
Jacobs C. (ed): Cancers of the Head and Neck. 1987. ISBN 0-89838-825-2.
MacDonald J.S. (ed): Gastrointestinal Oncology. 1987. ISBN 0-89838-829-5.
Ratliff T.L., Catalona W.J. (eds): Genitourinary Cancer. 1987. ISBN 0-89838-830-9.
Nathanson L. (ed): Basic and Clinical Aspects of Malignant Melanoma. 1987. ISBN 0-89838-856-2.
Muggia F.M. (ed): Concepts, Clinical Developments, and Therapeutic Advances in Cancer Chemotherapy.
1987. ISBN 0-89838-879-5.
Lippman, M.E., Dickson, R., (eds): Breast Cancer: Molecular and Cellular Biology. 1988.
ISBN 0-89838-368-4.
Osborne, C.K. (ed) Endocrine Therapies in Breast and Prostate Cancer. 1988. ISBN 0-89838-365-X.
Nathanson L. (ed): Malignant Melanoma: Biology, Diagnosis, a and Therapy. 1988. ISBN 0-89838-384-6.
Kamps W.A., Humphrey G.B., Poppema S. (eds): Hodgkin's Disease in Children. 1988. ISBN 0-89838-372-2.

Treatment of Soft Tissue Sarcomas

Edited by

HERBERT M. PINEDO

Department of Medical Oncology
Free University Hospital
Amsterdam, The Netherlands

and

JAAP VERWEIJ

Department of Medical Oncology
Rotterdam Cancer Institute
Rotterdam, The Netherlands

1989 **KLUWER ACADEMIC PUBLISHERS**
BOSTON / DORDRECHT / LONDON

Distributors for North America:
Kluwer Academic Publishers
101 Philip Drive
Assinippi Park
Norwell, Massachusetts 02061 USA

Distributors for the UK and Ireland:
Kluwer Academic Publishers
Falcon House, Queen Square
Lancaster LA1 1RN, UNITED KINGDOM

Distributors for all other countries:
Kluwer Academic Publishers Group
Distribution Centre
Post Office Box 322
3300 AH Dordrecht, THE NETHERLANDS

Library of Congress Cataloging-in-Publication Data

Treatment of soft tissue sarcomas / editors, H.M. Pinedo, J. Verweij.
   p. cm. —— (Cancer treatment and research)
  Includes bibliographies and index.
  ISBN 0-89838-391-9
  1. Sarcoma—Treatment. I. Pinedo, H.M. II. Verweij. J. (Jaap)
III. Series.
  [DNLM: 1. Sarcoma—therapy. 2. Soft Tissue Neoplasms—therapy.
W1 CA693 / WD 375 T784]
RC270.8.T75 1988
616.99'406—dc19
DNLM/DLC
for Library of Congress   88-12884
                                                CIP

PRINTED IN THE UNITED STATES OF AMERICA

Contents

Cancer Treatment and Research

Foreword

Where do you begin to look for a recent, authoritative article on the diagnosis or management of a particular malignancy? The few general oncology textbooks are generally out of date. Single papers in specialized journals are informative but seldom comprehensive; these are more often preliminary reports on a very limited number of patients. Certain general journals frequently publish good in-depth reviews of cancer topics, and published symposium lectures are often the best overviews available. Unfortunately, these reviews and supplements appear sporadically, and the reader can never be sure when a topic of special interest will be covered.

Cancer Treatment and Research is a series of authoritative volumes that aim to meet this need. It is an attempt to establish a critical mass of oncology literature covering virtually all oncology topics, revised frequently to keep the coverage up to date, easily available on a single library shelf or by a single personal subscription.

We have approached the problem in the following fashion: first, by dividing the oncology literature into specific subdivisions such as lung cancer, genitourinary cancer, and pediatric oncology; second, by asking eminent authorities in each of these areas to edit a volume on the specific topic on an annual or biannual basis. Each topic and tumor type is covered in a volume appearing frequently and predictably, discussing current diagnosis, staging, markers, all forms of treatment modalities, basic biology, and more.

In *Cancer Treatment and Research*, we have an outstanding group of editors, each having made a major commitment to bring to this new series the very best literature in his or her field. Kluwer Academic Publishers has made an equally major commitment to the rapid publication of high-quality books, and worldwide distribution.

Where can you go to find quickly a recent authoritative article on any major oncology problem? We hope that Cancer Treatment and Research provides an answer.

WILLIAM L. McGUIRE
Series Editor

Preface

One of the major advances of the last decade concerning the treatment of patients with soft tissue sarcomas is that an increased number of patients are being discussed in multidisciplinary teams prior to the initial treatment. The present volume on soft tissue sarcomas in the series *Cancer Treatment and Research* reflects the multidisciplinary approach with a focus on recent developments.

The availability of new histopathologic techniques has reduced the number of unclassified sarcomas and has furhter increased the importance of the histopathologist in providing estimates of the prognosis of the patient as well as data for the planning of treatment strategy. Further data for this strategy will be provided by diagnostic imaging. In this field, the role of magnetic resonance imaging has been further defined. Of utmost importance is the recent trend toward consensus in staging. The modification of the staging system of the American Joint Commission for Cancer Staging and End Results Reporting brings the possibility of a single staging system within reach in the next decade.

As surgery still provides the only chance for cure, the importance of being the most sparing as possible is obvious. For this reason, radiotherapy has been applied with success. The introduction of relatively new radiation techniques is therefore being observed with interest.

As for staging, there is also growing consensus about the role of chemotherapy in advanced disease. More and more trials have addressed the activity of the few truly active drugs, the most important being doxorubicin, ifosfamide and dacarbazine (DTIC). The answer to the question of whether single-agent chemotherapy is as effective as combination chemotherapy may be answered in the next few years. The lack of efficacy of adjuvant chemotherapy with the drugs presently available has definitively been demonstrated. Chemotherapy, however, may have an important role in the preoperative treatment of soft tissue sarcomas, although the optimal method of administration has yet to be defined.

A new topic in the present volume is thermochemotherapy, a combined-modality treatment with interesting preliminary results. Although the present volume focuses on new developments, previously obtained data are also briefly reviewed. With this in mind, we have invited a number of new authors to contribute to the present volume in order to extend its scope with regard to the present state of the art. We would like to thank all authors for their contributions.

H.M. Pinedo
J. Verweij

Contributing Authors

BRAMWELL, VIVIEN H.C., London Regional Cancer Centre, 391 South Street, London, Ontario N6A 4G5, Canada

BUTTINI, G.L., Department of Surgical Oncology, Regina Elena Cancer Institute, Via Regina Elena 291, 00161 Rome, Italy

CALABRO, A.M., Department of Surgical Oncology, Regina Elena Cancer Institute, Via Regina Elena 291, 00161 Rome, Italy

CARLINI, S., Department of Surgical Oncology, Regina Elena Cancer Institute, Via Regina Elena 291, 00161 Rome, Italy

CAVALLARI, A., Department of Surgical Oncology, Regina Elena Cancer Institute, Via Regina Elena 291, 00161 Rome, Italy

CAVALIERE, F., Department of Surgical Oncology, Regina Elena Cancer Institute, Via Regina Elena 291, 00161 Rome, Italy

CAVALIERE, R., Department of Surgical Oncology, Regina Elena Cancer Institute, Via Regina Elena 291, 00161 Rome, Italy

DI FILIPPO, F., Department of Surgical Oncology, Regina Elena Cancer Institute, Via Regina Elena 292, 00161 Rome, Italy

EILBER, FREDERICK R., Division of Oncology, Department of Surgery, UCLA School of Medicine, Los Angeles, CA 90024, U.S.A.

ENNEKING, WILLIAM F., Department of Orthopedics College of Medicine, University of Florida, Box J. 246, JHM Health Center, Gainesville, FL 32610, U.S.A.

FISHER, CYRIL, Department of Histopathology, Royal Marsden Hospital, Fulham Road, London SW3 6JJ, United Kingdom

GIANARELLI, D., Medical Physics and Expert Systems, Regina Elena Cancer Institute, Via Regina Elena 291, 00161 Rome, Italy

GRAZIANO, F., Department of Surgical Oncology, Regina Elena Cancer Institute, Via Regina Elena 291, 00161 Rome, Italy

GOLDING, RICHARD P., Department of Radiology, Free University Hospital, De Boelelaan 1117, 1081 HV Amsterdam, The Netherlands

GROENINGEN, CEES J., VAN, Department of Medical Oncology, Free University Hospital, De Boelelaan 1117, 1081 HV Amsterdam, The Netherlands

HUTH, JAMES F., Division of Oncology, Department of Surgery, UCLA School of Medicine, Los Angeles, CA 90024, U.S.A.

MOSCARELLI, F., Department of Surgical Oncology, Regina Elena Cancer Institute, Via Regina Elena 291, 00161 Rome, Italy

PINEDO, HERBERT M., Department of Medical Oncology, Free University Hospital, De Boelelaan 1117, 1081 HV Amsterdam, The Netherlands

SUIT, HERMAN, D., Department of Radiation Medicine, Massachusetts General Hospital Cancer Center, Harvard Medical School, Boston, MA 02114, U.S.A.

VALK, JAAP, Department of Radiology, Free University Hospital, De Boelelaan 1117, 1081 HV Amsterdam, The Netherlands

VERWEIJ, JAAP, Department of Medical Oncology, Rotterdam Cancer Institute, Groene Hilledijk 301, 3075 EA Rotterdam, The Netherlands

WESTBURY, G., Department of Surgery, Royal Marsden Hospital, Fulham Road, London SW3 6JJ, United Kingdom

VAN ZANTEN, THEA E.G., Department of Radiology, Free University Hospital, De Boelelaan 1117, 1081 HV Amsterdam, The Netherlands

Abbreviations

ADIC	=	Adriamycin (doxorubicin)–DTIC
AIDS	=	acquired immune deficiency syndrome
AJC	=	American Joint Commission for Cancer Staging and End Results Reporting
CAP	=	Cytoxan (cyclophosphamide), Adriamycin (doxorubicin), CDDP (Platinol)
CDDP	=	cisplatin (*cis*-diammine dichloroplatin)
CR	=	complete remission
CT	=	computer tomography
CTX	=	Cytoxan (cyclophosphamide)
CYVADIC	=	cyclophosphamide/vincristine/Adriamycin (doxorubicin)/DTIC
DACT	=	dactinomycin (actinomycin D)
DSA	=	digital subtraction angiography
DTIC	=	dacarbazine
DX	=	doxorubicin
ECOG	=	Eastern Cooperative Oncology Group
EORTC	=	European Organisation on Treatment and Research of Cancer
G	=	grade
GOG	=	Gynaecologic Oncology Group
HAP	=	hyperthermic antiblastic perfusion
i.a.	=	intra-arterial
IFOS	=	ifosfamide
i.v.	=	intravenous
LPAM	=	L-phenylalanine mustard (melphalan)
M	=	metastasis
MDR	=	multidrug resistance phenotype
MFH	=	malignant fibrous histiocytoma
MPNST	=	malignant peripheral nerve sheath tumor
MMS	=	mixed mesodermal sarcoma
MR	=	magnetic resonance
MTS	=	Musculoskeletal Tumor Society
NCI	=	National Cancer Institute

PR   = partial remission
OS   = overall survival
RFS   = relapse-free survival
SWOG   = Southwest Oncology Group
T   = tumor
VCR   = vincristine
VP-16   = etoposide
VRN   = von Recklinghausen's neurofibromatosis

TREATMENT OF SOFT TISSUE SARCOMAS

1. Pathology of soft tissue sarcomas

Cyril Fisher

Soft tissue sarcomas are a relatively rare type of primary malignant neoplasm, comprising <1% of all malignant tumors. They are a heterogeneous group of tumors with a wide range of biological behavior. They are grouped together on an anatomical basis and present common clinical problems that, together with the rarity of many of the subtypes, dictate a uniform clinicopathological approach. Nonetheless, accurate histopathological diagnosis is essential for management because the grading of soft tissue sarcomas is an integral part of most current staging systems and may be the most important single prognostic factor. Several studies [1–3] have emphasized that, for many sarcomas, prognosis is related directly to the diagnosis, i.e., the precise histological subtype. Thus, synovial sarcoma, epithelioid sarcoma, and rhabdomyosarcoma generally have a poor outlook. Other sarcomas, including many liposarcomas, leiomyosarcomas, nerve sheath tumors, and malignant fibrous histiocytomas have a wider spectrum of behavior and, in grading each case, microscopic details such as cellularity, pleomorphism, amount of necrosis, and mitotic count must be considered.

The basic histological patterns [4] of soft tissue sarcomas are familiar, but this group of tumors still retains considerable diagnostic difficulties for the pathologist. Some sarcomas, such as liposarcoma or rhabdomyosarcoma, resemble embryonic or adult mesenchymal-derived tissues and are readily identified. Others, for example, malignant fibrous histiocytoma and synovial sarcoma, do not have normal counterparts and often manifest a variety of histological patterns. Conversely, different sarcoma subtypes can share common microscopic appearances; a spindle cell morphology can be displayed by synovial sarcoma, leiomyosarcoma, malignant tumors of nerve sheath, rhabdomyosarcoma, malignant fibrous histiocytoma, and the (now rare) true fibrosarcoma. Round cell tumors include Ewing's sarcoma, rhabdomyosarcoma, neuroblastoma and epithelioid sarcoma, and on occasion these require distinction from lymphoma, melanoma, and carcinoma.

Diagnosis depends on the detection of specific features of cellular differentiation, which may not be apparent in ordinary histological sections. The supplementary techniques of immunohistochemistry, electron microscopy, and cytogenetics can often reveal such differentiation in soft tissue sarcomas;

Pinedo, H.M., Verweij, J., eds. TREATMENT OF SOFT TISSUE SARCOMAS.
© Kluwer Academic Publishers, Boston. ISBN: 0-89838-391-9. All rights reserved.

this not only results in increased accuracy of diagnosis, but has suggested new concepts of histogenesis and challenged established nomenclature. This chapter reviews recent pathological observations for the main sarcoma subtypes, and considers current concepts of grading soft tissue sarcomas.

Classification and frequency

Using standard nomenclature [4], the distribution of diagnoses in a consecutive series of 200 soft tissue sarcomas studied at the Royal Marsden Hospital, London, is shown in Table 1. Malignant fibrous histiocytoma is the commonest category, and fibrosarcoma, if strictly defined (see below), is extremely uncommon. There was no evidence of differentiation by light or electron microscopy or by immunohistochemistry in 3.5% of tumors, and these remain uncategorized.

Malignant fibrous histiocytoma

Malignant fibrous histiocytoma (MFH) is the adult soft tissue sarcoma diagnosed most frequently today. The category now includes many tumors previously considered as fibrosarcoma, pleomorphic rhabdomyosarcoma, or

Table 1. Distribution of 200 sarcomas diagnosed by light and electron microscopy and immunohistochemistry

Diagnosis	No. of cases	(%)
Malignant fibrous histiocytoma	57	(28.5)
Liposarcoma	38	(19)
Rhabdomyosarcoma	26	(13)
Synovial sarcoma	21	(10.5)
Malignant nerve sheath tumor	12	(6)
Extraskeletal osseous tumors	11	(5.5)
Ewing's sarcoma	5	
Chondrosarcoma	3	
Osteosarcoma	3	
Epithelioid sarcoma	7	(3.5)
Leiomyosarcoma	7	(3.5)
Myofibrosarcoma and fibrosarcoma	4	(2)
Fibrosarcoma	1	
Angiosarcoma	4	(2)
Malignant hemangiopericytoma	1	(0.5)
Alveolar soft part sarcoma	3	(1.5)
Clear cell sarcoma	2	(1)
Unclassified	7	(3.5)
Total	200	(100)

undifferentiated pleomorphic sarcoma. While occurring most frequently in the extremities and retroperitoneum, MFH can involve any part of the body [5]. The wide range of histological patterns within this entity includes storiform-pleomorphic, myxoid [6], inflammatory [7], and angiomatoid [8] variants as well as malignant giant cell tumor of soft parts [9]. In general, the tumors are of intermediate or high grade with size and depth from surface being important additional prognostic factors [10]; the relatively few cases arising superficial to the deep fascia have a good prognosis [5]. Some regard dermatofibrosarcoma protuberans as a superficial MFH, and atypical fibroxanthoma has also been included in this category [4].

MFH was originally designated malignant fibroxanthoma [11]. Tissue culture studies [12] had suggested origin from histiocytes that, it was thought, could behave as facultative fibroblasts. Ultrastructurally, cells with characteristics of histiocytes, of fibroblasts, of both, and of their supposed derivatives (giant cells, myofibroblasts) have been observed [13–16] as well as primitive (supposedly stem) cells. Although of diagnostic use, the lack of specificity of these morphological observations limits their contribution to determining the nature of the tumor. The immunohistochemical detection of alpha-1-antitrypsin and alpha-1-antichymotrypsin supported the hypothesis of histiocytic differentiation [17, 18]. These enzymes were regarded initially as markers for histiocytes, but are now known to be detectable in a variety of other tumors [19], although they remain of use in diagnosing MFH in the appropriate histological context. However, the concept of the histiocytic nature of MFH has been challenged by recent studies with cell type-specific antibodies which showed [20–23] that most markers for cells of monocyte/macrophage lineage were absent from the tumor cells. These immunohistochemical [22, 23] studies, together with enzyme histochemical [22] data, have demonstrated a fibroblastic phenotype, suggesting that this tumor originates from primitive mesenchymal cells rather than histiocytes. The monoclonal antibodies to monocytes/macrophages used in these studies recognize marrow-derived cells, and the histiocyte-like cells in MFH may be of a different lineage. Some cases of MFH have in fact demonstrated monocyte/macrophage markers [20, 24], but this is not necessarily inconsistent with the concept of origin from locally derived pluripotential primitive cells.

Support for this concept has come from the demonstration in MFH of coexpression of intermediate filament subtypes. All MFHs, in common with other mesenchymal tumors, display vimentin and, in some, desmin has been demonstrated, perhaps correlating with myofibroblastic differentiation. The additional expression of neurofilament and cytokeratin [25] in ultrastructurally confirmed cases of these tumors suggests multidirectional differentiation in mesenchymal cells. MFH can arise in, or be associated with, other types of sarcoma and it has been postulated [26] that MFH, representing a dedifferentiated stage, is a final common pathway for other soft tissue sarcomas.

Diagnosis of MFH is usually possible by routine light microscopy. Distinction of pleomorphic tumors from rhabdomyosarcoma can be made utilizing myoglobin immunohistochemistry, and from liposarcoma occasionally by electron microscopy [27, 28].

Liposarcoma

Liposarcomas are classified by histological appearance into well-differentiated, myxoid, round cell, and pleomorphic types, the first two having a good prognosis and the last two being of high grade [29–32]. It has been suggested [33, 34] that well-differentiated liposarcoma of the extremities (but not of the retroperitoneum) should, because of its excellent prognosis, be reclassified as an atypical lipoma.

The relatively distinctive morphology of liposarcoma, which includes the presence of lipoblasts, means that special diagnostic techniques are rarely required. Pleomorphic liposarcoma can be difficult to distinguish from pleomorphic malignant fibrous histiocytoma, especially as some lipid may be found in cells of the latter, and electron microscopy is sometimes useful here [27]. Electron microscopy can also help in the diagnosis of those myxoid liposarcomas from which typical lipoblasts are absent; primitive lipoblasts often have an external lamina that is absent from the cells of MFH [35, 36]. Some liposarcomas demonstrate S100 protein [37]; this is unlikely to be a source of diagnostic confusion with nerve sheath tumors, and may assist in distinguishing myoxid liposarcoma from myxoid malignant fibrous histiocytoma [38].

A consistent chromosomal translocation, t(12;16), has been reported in myxoid liposarcoma [39].

Rhabdomyosarcoma

The three major histological subtypes of rhabdomyosarcoma characterized by skeletal muscle differentiation are embryonal, alveolar, and pleomorphic [4].

Most interest has centered on the recognition of childhood embryonal rhabdomyosarcomas. Those composed of small cells are likely to be confused with other similar tumors (Ewing's sarcoma, neuroblastoma, and lymphoma); these are myoglobin negative. Alveolar rhabdomyosarcoma is not difficult to diagnose histologically, and pleomorphic rhabdomyosarcoma, occurring in adults, has become a rare tumor since the recognition that many cases previously so identified are in fact liposarcomas or malignant fibrous histiocytomas.

The immunohistochemical demonstration of specific or semispecific markers for muscle differentiation has made the diagnosis of rhabdomyosarcoma much easier. Myoglobin, which is specific for skeletal (and cardiac) muscle, is demonstrable in 60%–90% of embryonal rhabdomyosarcomas [40–43] and in all alveolar and pleomorphic rhabdomyosarcomas [41]. In embryonal tumors, however, myoglobin is detectable only in cells with a sufficient amount of cytoplasm. Desmin is demonstrable in many embryonal rhabdomyosarcomas [44], although the reported sensitivity of its detection varies between 50% [45]

and 100% [46]. This intermediate filament is also present in smooth muscle, but the morphological and clinical differences from rhabdomyosarcoma should prevent confusion. Furthermore, the other histologically similar tumors of childhood lack desmin. Other markers advocated for diagnosis of rhabdomyosarcoma include myosin, which appears to be less sensitive than desmin [47], creatine kinase [48], beta-enolase [49], and Z protein [50], but none of these has been sufficiently assessed for specificity in routine diagnostic use.

Skeletal muscle differentiation is characterized ultrastructurally by the presence of thick and thin intermediate filaments with or without Z-band formation [51]. Unfortunately, such features can be detected in only about half of all embryonal rhabdomyosarcomas [52], and therefore electron microscopy has less to offer than immunohistochemistry in this area. Kahn et al. [48] compared electron microscopy with immunohistochemistry and found that only 37% of childhood embryonal rhabdomyosarcomas were myoglobin positive, whereas 54% of the cases examined showed the characteristic ultrastructure. In a study at the Royal Marsden Hospital, London, 13 (76%) of 17 embryonal rhabdomyosarcomas displayed myoglobin positivity, whereas only 8 (47%) could be diagnosed by electron microscopy.

A consistent chromosomal translocation, t(2;13), has been demonstrated in examples of alveolar rhabdomyosarcoma [53].

Malignant peripheral nerve sheath tumors

About 12% of soft tissue sarcomas show nerve sheath differentiation; they may arise in recognizable nerve trunks, in neurofibromas, or without any discernible nervous connection. Since they are not always composed of Schwann cells or of fibroblasts, and since they may be considered to be of neuroectodermal origin, the term malignant peripheral nerve sheath tumor (MPNST) [54] is preferable to malignant schwannoma or neurofibrosarcoma, unless the cellular composition has been demonstrated by immunohistochemistry and electron microscopy. About half of these tumors are associated with von Recklinghausen's neurofibromatosis (VRN) [55], in which there is at least a 5% chance of malignant change. The rest are sporadic, although the incidence of these may be somewhat higher than generally reported, as a number of cases without obvious neural origin are, without electron microscopy, incorrectly diagnosed as fibrosarcoma or MFH [56]. Histological patterns include a spindle cell type with characteristic nuclear morphology, a rare epithelioid variant resembling melanoma or carcinoma [57], and a pleomorphic MFH-like tumor seen more frequently complicating VRN. Heterotopic epithelial or cartilaginous metaplasia is occasionally seen [58, 59] and a skeletal muscle component is present in the high-grade triton tumor [60–63].

Ultrastructurally, nerve sheath tumors may be shown to be composed of two major cell types, the Schwann cell (Fig. 1) and the perineurial cell (Fig. 2) [54, 64, 65] although most authors [66–70] have sought or recognized only Schwann cells. Both types are present in some neurofibromas, but in a per-

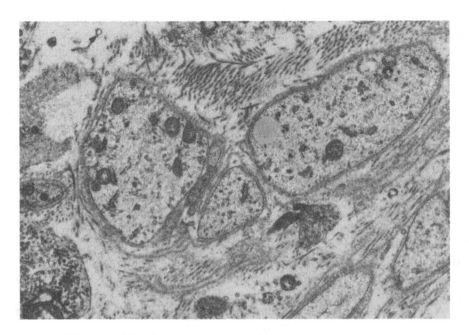

Figure 1. Malignant peripheral nerve sheath tumor. Electron micrograph showing Schwann cell differentiation. Transected cell processes have continuous external lamina, reduplicated layers of which are seen in the stroma. ×20,000.

sonally studied series of 16 cases of MPNSTs, one cell type was usually predominant. Electron-microscopic evidence of Schwann cell differentiation, with interdigitating cytoplasmic processes, junctions, and external lamina (Fig. 1) is seen in ~50% of cases, albeit in some poorly developed with loss of external lamina. Others show features of perineurial cells, which are bipolar with long processes displaying prominent pinocytosis, fragmented external lamina, and tight junctions [54, 64, 65] (Fig. 2). Transitional forms occur between these two cell types, and between perineurial cells and fibroblasts, and transitions to melanoma have been reported [71, 72]. The pleomorphic tumors arising in VRN ultrastructurally resemble MFH.

Immunohistochemical positivity for S100 protein is seen in tumors with Schwann cell differentiation, but not in those composed of other cell types [64, 70]. Thus, only 50%–70% of MPNSTs display S100 protein [73–75]. When positive, this is of diagnostic value, since S100 protein is absent from the other spindle cell sarcomas with which this tumor is likely to be confused (fibrosarcoma, synovial sarcoma). More recently, anti-Leu-7 (HNK1), a monoclonal antibody recognizing lymphocytes with killer cell functions [76] that also reacts with a myelin-associated glycoprotein [77], has been detected in some S100-negative MPNSTs [78]; it was not detected in fibrosarcomas. Its presence in leiomyosarcoma and synovial sarcoma [79] restricts its use in sarcoma diagnosis to forming part of a panel of antibodies. Nerve sheath tumors

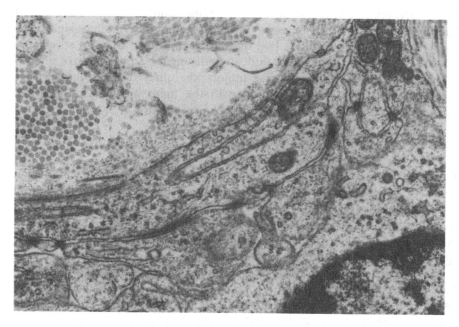

Figure 2. Malignant peripheral nerve sheath tumor. Electron micrograph shows long processes interdigitating, with tight intercellular junctions and pinocytosis, but no continuous external lamina. These resemble the processes of perineurial cells. ×32,000.

contain vimentin and occasionally glial fibrillary acidic protein [80], but the reported presence of desmin in some MPNSTs [78] requires confirmation.

Leiomyosarcoma

Leiomyosarcoma occurs most commonly in the retroperitoneum, and in the skin and subcutaneous tissues, but occasionally arises in the deep soft tissues of the limbs. The microscopic appearance of smooth muscle, with fascicles of spindle cells with blunt-ended nuclei, pale eosinophilic cytoplasm, and little intercellular collagen, is obvious in well-differentiated leiomyosarcomas, but in the less well differentiated tumors distinction from other spindle cell sarcomas and sometimes from pleomorphic MFH may be necessary. The intermediate filament desmin, the marker for muscle differentiation, is found in >50% [45, 83–86] of leiomyosarcomas although it may not be detectable in poorly differentiated examples [87], where its demonstration would be of most value. Also, desmin is not completely specific, since it can be seen in some cells of MFH [25]. The absence of S100 protein and of epithelial markers enables distinction from MPNST and monophasic synovial sarcoma, respectively.

The electron microscope can show features of smooth muscle differentiation; these include myofilaments with dense bodies, plasmalemmal thickenings, micropinocytosis, intercellular junctions, and formation of external lamina. Again, caution is necessary in interpreting these findings since they can be seen in myofibroblasts [88] that are found in a variety of soft tissue tumors [14, 16], and that may be difficult to distinguish from primitive smooth muscle cells. As with all soft tissue tumors, the ultrastructural observations must be interpreted in conjunction with the light microscopy, including immunohistochemical findings, and the clinical picture.

Vascular tumors

Angiosarcomas are found most commonly in the skin and subcutis of the head and neck of older people, where they are tumors of poor prognosis, with an overall 5-year survival of 30%–75% [89, 90]. They also arise in breast [91] and liver, and occasionally in deep soft tissues including the limbs and retroperitoneum [4]. The histological appearances vary from well-formed vascular spaces to those of spindle or round cell sarcoma, and in these cases positivity for Factor VIII-related antigen [92–94] or for *Ulex* lectin [95, 96] will confirm the vascular endothelial nature of the tumor. These cells have a characteristic ultrastructure [89], with tight junctions, pinocytosis, and Weibel-Palade bodies, although the latter are often difficult to find in angiosarcomas.

Epithelioid hemangioendothelioma is a recently described [97] low-grade tumor arising in any site (usually skin), and often associated with a large blood vessel, in which polygonal, vacuolated tumor cells are arranged in cords in a fibrous stroma. Positivity for Factory VIII-related antigen [98] and *Ulex*, and absence of epithelial markers, distinguish this lesion from metastatic carcinoma, which it otherwise resembles.

Kaposi's sarcoma is a vascular tumor of the skin that has aroused recent interest because of its association with acquired immune deficiency syndrome (AIDS). The classic form is sporadic and affects the lower extremities of older men as an indolent tumor, although eventual visceral dissemination occurs in many cases. The endemic form occurs in Africa in younger patients; lymph node involvement may occur. In AIDS cases, the clinical picture is similar, although head and neck involvement occurs and the disease spreads to internal organs. Histologically [99], early lesions show a nondescript focal vascular and inflammatory proliferation. Later lesions have more spindle cells with intercellular slits containing blood, and may resemble fibrosarcoma or angiosarcoma. Vascular endothelial markers are found in some [100] but not all tumor cells, and pericytes and fibroblasts may also be present [101].

The prognosis is extremely variable, and spontaneous regression has been recorded [102]. The neoplastic nature of Kaposi's sarcoma has been questioned [101].

Hemangiopericytoma [103] is a tumor of uncertain nature. Pericytomatous patterns can be seen in many sarcomas, particularly synovial, and the presence of any marker excludes hemangiopericytoma. Some marker-negative cases have partial smooth muscle differentiation (personal observations).

Fibrosarcoma

The incidence of fibrosarcoma has diminished in recent times, due partly to the recognition of malignant fibrous histiocytoma and partly to more accurate diagnosis of other histologically similar spindle cell sarcomas such as monophasic synovial sarcoma and malignant peripheral nerve sheath tumor as a result of immunohistochemical methods. Indeed, if strictly defined as a marker-negative (except for vimentin) tumor composed only of cells with the ultrastructural morphology of fibroblasts, fibrosarcoma is extremely rare: only one example was found in a series of 200 soft tissue sarcomas subjected to electron microscopy by the author. Some fibroblastic sarcomas also have focal or widespread myofibroblastic differentiation, but fall short of the full electron-microscopic picture of smooth muscle. These are usually uniform spindle cell tumors, lacking desmin, and may be termed myofibrosarcomas. Such sarcomas, together with fibrosarcoma, account for only 2% of the tumors in the author's series (Table 1). Among sarcomas, there are recent indications, however, that the diagnostic pendulum may swing back with ultrastructural [104] and immunohistochemical [20, 22] evidence supporting the fibroblastic nature of some malignant fibrous histiocytomas.

It should be borne in mind that, in some series, published figures for behavior and retrospective grading of soft tissue sarcomas may be inaccurate to the extent that fibrosarcoma has been overdiagnosed.

Fibromatosis, which is not usually regarded as a sarcoma since it may recur locally but does not metastasize, is composed of active fibroblasts, but often also shows focal myofibroblastic differentiation.

Synovial sarcoma

Synovial sarcoma is a tumor predominantly of young adults that arises in soft tissues around large joints, particularly the knee, although its occurrence within a joint is rare. Characteristically, this is a biphasic tumor with spindle cell and epithelial-like areas, in varying proportion. The spindle cells are closely packed and rather uniform with little cytoplasm and, when the epithelial component is minimal or lacking, monophasic synovial sarcoma can be distinguished from other spindle cell sarcomas by careful light-microscopic examination. The monophasic epithelial pattern is extremely rare, and must be distinguished from epithelioid sarcoma. The existence of monophasic forms of the tumor was disputed, but has now been confirmed by the demonstration of the epithelial markers keratin [105–107] and epithelial membrane antigen [107] not only in the epithelial component but also in the spindle cells of this tumor. One or other marker is present in some spindle cells of at least 80% of cases. In addition, electron microscopy (Fig. 3) shows that, whereas the epithelial structures have features of adenocarcinoma, the spindle cells of both biphasic and monophasic tumors have focal incomplete glandular differentiation with microvillous or filopodial processes protruding into intercellular

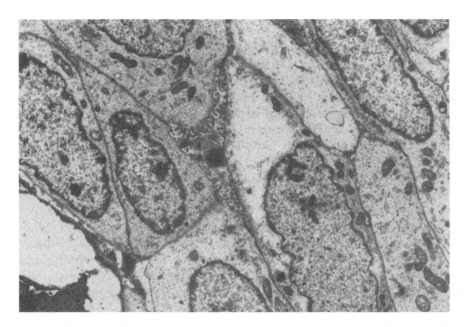

Figure 3. Synovial sarcoma, spindle component. Electron micrograph shows intercellular spaces into which project microvilli, with junctions between adjacent cells. This is regarded as attempted epithelial differentiation. ×7500.

spaces with junctional specializations [107–109]. The ultrastructure may be diagnostic in marker-negative cases [107]. Thus, synovial sarcoma is unique among spindle cell sarcomas in demonstrating epithelial differentiation. Furthermore, the status of this tumor as a discrete entity has been confirmed by the demonstration in all cases so far examined of a specific and consistent chromosomal translocation, t(x;18) [110, 111]. It is clear that synovial sarcoma is not related to synovium, in origin or in direction of differentiation, and its designation has been questioned [112].

The prognosis of synovial sarcoma has been regarded as poor, with 5-year survival of 25%–50%, but there is evidence of improvement with modern methods of management [113]. The histological pattern may affect outcome [109, 114, 115] although no recent large series has taken into account the newer concepts of this tumor, which will alter its apparent incidence. The calcifying variant has a better prognosis [116].

Epithelioid sarcoma

Epithelioid sarcoma [117, 118] is a tumor arising most commonly in the extremities of young adults, forming centrally necrotic nodules of deceptively bland-looking plump epithelioid cells that are often misdiagnosed at initial presentation, as a granuloma or as melanoma, carcinoma, or even rhabdomyosarcoma. It is, however, of high-grade malignancy with frequent local recurrence and eventual metastasis. Like synovial sarcoma, this tumor shows epithelial differentiation. Cytokeratin can be demonstrated in some [118, 119] or all [120–122] cases, as can epithelial membrane antigen [121–123] as well as the intermediate filament vimentin, enabling distinction from the other conditions. Electron microscopy has helped to reconcile the conflicting theories of the origin of this tumor by showing a spectrum of differentiation from primitive or fibrohistiocytic cells (some myofibroblastic) to those resembling carcinoma cells with full epithelial differentiation evidenced by intercellular junctions, surface microvilli, tonofilaments, and external lamina [122]. Most cases show partial epithelial differentiation, with similarities to synovial sarcoma. Nonetheless, there ae sufficient differences [118] to conclude that, while some cases of epithelioid sarcoma are variants of synovial sarcoma, most are not.

A cultured cell line has been established from an epithelioid sarcoma and its characteristics and cytogenetic constitution described [124].

Clear cell sarcoma

Typically arising in the extremities (particularly the lower leg) of young adults [125, 126], clear cell sarcoma is characterized by well-defined nests of cells with clear or eosinophilic cytoplasm. It is a high-grade tumor likely to recur and metastasize. Although it has been regarded [127] as part of the spectrum of tendosynovial sarcoma, clear cell sarcoma lacks epithelial markers. Instead, over half of these tumors contain stainable melanin, with melanosomes found by electron microscopy, and S100 protein positivity has been demonstrated in the majority of cases examined [128–130]. These observations indicate a neural crest origin for the tumor, and its redesignation as malignant melanoma of soft parts has been suggested [129]. An account of the ultrastructure has shown a relationship to nerve sheath tumor [131].

Alveolar soft part sarcoma

This entity [132] is composed of nests of loosely cohesive large cells somewhat resembling renal cell carcinoma, with abundant cytoplasm that contains striking, periodic acid–Schiff-positive crystalline material. This is membrane bound with a characteristic ultrastructure (Fig. 4), but is of unknown composition. A similarity to renin has been postulated [133], but not been confirmed, and digital image processing has suggested the filamentous structure of actin [134]. Theories about the nature of this tumor have included a modified smooth muscle, or neural or muscular histogenesis, based on the various demonstrations of renin [133], of neural structures [135], and of rhabdomyoma-like inclusions [136]. Recently, supportive evidence for a myogenic origin has come from the immunohistochemical demonstration in some cases of desmin and Z protein [137]. Myoglobin was not detected, but the skeletal muscle

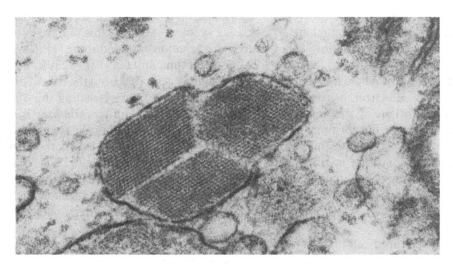

Figure 4. Alveolar soft part sarcoma. Electron micrograph of the characteristic membrane-bound crystalline structures. ×121,000.

enzyme beta-enolase was found biochemically. On the other hand, in a larger study, Auerbach and Brooks [138] (using antibodies thought unlikely to cross react with vimentin) could not demonstrate desmin positivity. Myoglobin was also lacking, and S100 protein and neuron-specific enolase were also not detected, providing no support for a neural crest origin. While it is possible that some alveolar soft part sarcomas show muscular differentiation, it is clear that the origin and nature of this tumor remain unknown. It is a high-grade sarcoma, occurring mainly in the lower limb of young adults, although head and neck tumors are found in children. Although slowly growing, metastasis eventually occurs in the majority of cases, with a 5-year survival of ~60% [139, 140].

Extraskeletal osseous sarcomas

Soft tissue chondrosarcoma, of conventional or myxoid (chordoid sarcoma) patterns, demonstrates S100 protein [141], but not epithelial markers, aiding a distinction from chordoma [142–144]. Electron microscopy may also be helpful here [145]. S100 protein is absent from the undifferentiated areas of mesenchymal chondrosarcoma [146]. Osteosarcoma of the soft tissues [147] has no specific cellular marker to enable distinction from other types of sarcoma with areas of ossification.

Tumors indistinguishable from Ewing's sarcoma of bone have been described in soft tissues [148–150] in children and, mainly, in young adults. They are composed of uniform round cells, typically containing abundant glycogen, and can present a problem of diagnosis from other round cell tumors of soft tissue. Ultrastructurally, the glycogen is confirmed and poorly formed intercellular junctions are regularly seen [151], but there are no specific features. The intercellular junctions have been reported to stain for desmoplakin [152], demonstrating their desmosomal nature. Immunohistochemically, lymphoid, muscle, and other epithelial markers are absent. Vimentin is the principal intermediate filament detected in the tumor cells [153] although recently keratin and neurofilament have also been described in a few cases [152], leading to the postulation that Ewing's sarcoma is a pluripotential or blastomatous neoplasm.

A specific chromosomal translocation, t(11; 22), has been described in Ewing's sarcoma of bone [154–156].

Grading

The prognosis and management of soft tissue sarcomas depend on staging, i.e., the extent of spread at the time of diagnosis. All staging systems [157] take into account the grade of a tumor. Grading is a histological term that usually relates to the degree of differentiation, i.e., resemblance to parent (adult-type) tissue. Its use lies in attempting to predict behavior by matching the appearances of a tumor with the accumulated experience of its natural history. For carcinomas, this is relatively easy since, in each case, we are dealing with a single distinct entity and know what it is trying to resemble. For sarcomas, the problem is more difficult because the term embraces many different types of mesenchymal tumor. Some resemble adult tissue, e.g., nerve sheath or smooth muscle tumors, yet may have a poor prognosis even when well differentiated. Others recapitulate normal embryonic tissue, but may have a good or a bad prognosis: although rhabdomyosarcomas are high grade, myxoid liposarcomas are not. Additionally, in many sarcomas, the concept of differentiation becomes problematic; some types, such as alveolar soft part sarcoma or epithelioid sarcoma, are always undifferentiated in the sense that they do not resemble any known normal adult tissue, and yet have a relatively consistent microscopic appearance.

The matter is simplified since some sarcomas always have a slow course and low metastatic potential, and others are always aggressive. The histological type (diagnosis) therefore can be used as an initial grading criterion, not necessarily related to differentiation, for placing tumors into a good or bad prognostic category. The drawbacks of this approach include [1] intraobserver variation: two studies [158, 159] found only 65% and 61% concordance for diagnosis with a mean of three diagnoses per case [158], although concordance for grading was 75% [159]. Also, in retrospective studies, without the benefit of immunohistochemistry and electron microscopy, the apparent frequency of each subtype may be incorrect. This is particularly so for the incidence of fibrosarcoma (see above) and of unclassified sarcomas.

Within other subtypes, there is a wider spectrum of behavior, and in these grading is an attempt to relate behavior to pathology. These include MFH, leiomyosarcoma, fibrosarcoma, and some liposarcomas, and each may require different histological criteria for grading. These have been assessed by various observers, some of whom apply them to all sarcomas and others only to those with a wider behavioral spectrum. Features used are mitotic counts, cellularity, differentiation/pleomorphism, and amount of necrosis. Different groups have found that, of these, the best predictors of prognosis were mitotic counts [160], mitoses and amount of necrosis [161], mitoses, necrosis and differentiation [162], mitoses, pleomorphism, and cellularity [163], or mitoses, cellularity, pleomorphism, vascularity, and necrosis [157]. One study, which graded some cases first by diagnosis, found that the amount of necrosis was the single major predictor for survival among the other tumors [2]. In all series, higher-grade tumors form a substantial majority.

Grading of tumors is an attempt to divide a continuum. As well as being necessarily arbitrary, this procedure may be affected by unrepresentative tumor sampling and by subjective variation [158, 159]. Perhaps for these reasons, there is no agreement on the optimum number of grades, nor on the extent to which diagnosis alone should be used as a grading criterion. At the two extremes, some centers now grade solely by diagnosis [3], forming three groups, while others insist that all cases should be graded by histological features irrespective of diagnosis. Among these, tumors have been assigned to one of two [164], three [157, 160, 165], or four [163, 166] grades according to various combinations of observations. Regrading by diagnosis of a group of sarcomas previously graded by histological features [3] led to reassignation of staging with apparent improvement of 2-year disease-free interval in earlier-stage cases.

It is evident that grading is an important prognostic factor, and it is desirable that uniformity of approach be attained. With the knowledge that some sarcomas are chromosomally distinct entities, it may be better to grade each tumor type on a separate basis, either by diagnosis or by histological features, rather than to apply a single schema to all sarcomas regardless of the differences among tumor types.

References

1. Russell WO, Cohen J, Enzinger F, Hajdu SI, Heise H, Martin RG, Meissner W, Miller WT, Schmitz RL, Suit HD: A clinical and pathological staging system for soft tissue sarcomas. Cancer 40:1562–1570, 1977.
2. Costa J, Wesley RA, Glatstein E, Rosenberg SA: The grading of soft tissue sarcomas: results of a clinicohistopathologic correlation in a series of 163 cases. Cancer 53:530–541, 1984.
3. Lindberg R: Treatment of localised soft tissue sarcomas in adults at MD Anderson Hospital and Tumor Institute (1960–1981). Cancer Treat Symp 3:59–65, 1985.
4. Enzinger FM, Weiss SW: Soft tissue tumors. St Louis: CV Mosby, 1983.
5. Weiss SW, Enzinger FM: Malignant fibrous histiocytoma: an analysis of 200 cases. Cancer 41:2250–2266, 1978.

6. Lagace R, Delage C, Seemayer TA: Myxoid variety of malignant fibrous histiocytoma: ultrastructural observations. Cancer 43:526–534, 1979.
7. Kyriacos M, Kempson RL: Inflammatory fibrous histiocytoma: an aggressive and lethal lesion. Cancer 37:1584–1606, 1976.
8. Enzinger FM: Angiomatoid malignant fibrous histiocytoma: a distinct fibrohistiocytic tumor of children and young adults simulating a vascular neoplasm. Cancer 44:2147–2157, 1979.
9. Guccion JG, Enzinger FM: Malignant giant cell tumor of soft parts: an analysis of 32 cases. Cancer 29:1518–1529, 1972.
10. Rydholm A, Syk I: Malignant fibrous histiocytoma of soft tissue: correlation between clinical variables and histologic malignancy grade. Cancer 57:2323–2324, 1986.
11. O'Brien JE, Stout AP: Malignant fibrous xanthomas. Cancer 17:1445–1455, 1964.
12. Ozello L, Stout AP, Murray MR: Cultural characteristics of malignant fibrous histiocytomas and fibrous xanthomas. Cancer 16:331–344, 1963.
13. FU Y-S, Gabbiani G, Kaye GI, Lattes R: Malignant soft tissue tumors of probable histiocytic origin (malignant fibrous histiocytomas): general considerations and electron microscopic and tissue culture studies. Cancer 35:176–198, 1975.
14. Churg AM, Kahn LB: Myofibroblasts and related cells in malignant fibrous and fibrohistiocytic tumors. Hum Pathol 8:205–218, 1977.
15. Harris M: The ultrastructure of benign and malignant fibrous histiocytomas. Histopathology 4:29–44, 1980.
16. Tsuneyoshi M, Enjoji M, Shinohara N: Malignant fibrous histiocytoma: an electron microscopic study of 17 cases. Virchows Arch [Pathol Anat] 392:135–145, 1981.
17. Kindblom L-G, Jacobsen GK, Jacobsen M: Immunohistochemical investigations of tumors of supposed fibroblastic–histiocytic origin. Hum Pathol 13:834–840, 1982.
18. Du Boulay CEH: Demonstration of alpha-1-antitrypsin and alpha-1-antichymotrypsin in fibrous histiocytomas using the immunoperoxidase technique. Am J Surg Pathol 6:559–564, 1982.
19. Leader M, Patel J, Collins M, Henry K: Anti-alpha 1-antichymotrypsin staining of 194 sarcomas, 38 carcinomas and 17 malignant melanomas: its lack of specificity as a tumor marker. Am J Surg Pathol 11:133–139, 1987.
20. Roholl PJM, Kleyne J, van Unnik JAM: Characterization of tumor cells in malignant fibrous histiocytomas and other soft tissue tumors, in comparison with malignant histiocytes. Am J Pathol 121:269–274, 1985.
21. Roholl PJM, Kleijne J, van Basten CDH, van der Putte SCJ, van Unnik JAM: A study to analyze the origin of tumor cells in malignant fibrous histiocytomas: a multiparametric characterization. Cancer 56:2809–2815, 1985.
22. Wood GS, Beckstead JH, Turner RR, Hendrickson MR, Kempson RL, Warnke RA: Malignant fibrous histiocytoma tumor cells resemble fibroblasts. Am J Surg Pathol 10: 323–335, 1986.
23. Brecher ME, Franklin WA: Absence of mononuclear phagocyte antigens in malignant fibrous histiocytoma. Am J Clin Pathol 86:344–348, 1986.
24. Strauchen JA, Dimitriu-Bona A: Malignant fibrous histiocytoma: expression of monocyte–macrophage differentiation antigens detected with monoclonal antibodies. Am J Pathol 124:303–309, 1986.
25. Lawson CW, Fisher C, Gatter KC: An immunohistochemical study of differentiation in malignant fibrous histiocytoma. Histopathology 11:375–383, 1987.
26. Brooks JJ: The significance of double phenotypic patterns and markers in human sarcomas: a new model of mesenchymal differentiation. Am J Pathol 125:113–123, 1986.
27. Reddick RL, Michelitch H, Triche TJ: Malignant soft tissue tumors (malignant fibrous histiocytoma, pleomorphic liposarcoma and pleomorphic rhabdomyosarcoma): an electron microscopic study. Hum Pathol 10:327–343, 1979.
28. Weiss LM, Warhol MJ: Ultrastructural distinctions between adult pleomorphic rhabdomyosarcomas, pleomorphic liposarcomas, and pleomorphic malignant fibrous histiocytomas. Hum Pathol 15:1025–1033, 1984.

29. Enterline HT, Culberson JD, Rochlin DB, Bradly LW: Liposarcoma: a clinical and pathological study of 53 cases. Cancer 13:932–950, 1960.
30. Enzinger FM, Winslow DJ: Liposarcoma: a study of 103 cases. Virchows Arch [Pathol Anat] 335:367–388, 1962.
31. Evans HL: Liposarcoma: a study of 55 cases with a reassessment of its classification. Am J Surg Pathol 3:507–523, 1979.
32. Orson GG, Sim FH, Reiman HM, Taylor WF: Liposarcoma of the musculoskeletal system. Cancer 60:1362–1370, 1987.
33. Evans HL, Soule EH, Winkelmann RK: Atypical lipoma, atypical intramuscular lipoma, and well-differentiated retroperitoneal liposarcoma: a reappraisal of 30 cases formerly classified as well-differentiated liposarcoma. Cancer 43:574–584, 1979.
34. Azumi N, Curtis J, Kempson RL, Hendrickson MR: Atypical and malignant neoplasms showing lipomatous differentiation: a study of 111 cases. Am J Surg Pathol 11:161–183, 1987.
35. Kindblom L-G, Save-Soderbergh J: The ultrastructure of liposarcoma: a study of 10 cases. Acta Pathol Microbiol Scand [A] 87:109–121, 1979.
36. Bolen JW, Thorning D: Benign lipoblastoma and myxoid liposarcoma: a comparative light- and electron-microscopic study. Am J Surg Pathol 4:163–174, 1980.
37. Cocchia D, Lauriola L, Stolfi VM, Tallini G, Michetti F: S100 antigen labels neoplastic cells in liposarcoma and cartilaginous tumors. Virchows Arch [Pathol Anat] 403:139–145, 1983.
38. Hashimoto H, Daimaru Y, Enjoji M: S-100 protein distribution in liposarcoma: an immunoperoxidase study with special reference to the distinction of liposarcomas from myxoid malignant fibrous histiocytoma. Virchows Arch [Pathol Anat] 405:1–10, 1984.
39. Limon J, Turc-Carel C, Dal Cin P, Rao U, Sandberg AA: Recurrent chromosome translocations in liposarcoma. Cancer Genet Cytogenet 22:93–94, 1986.
40. Corson JM, Pinkus GS: Intracellular myoglobin: a specific marker for skeletal muscle differentiation in soft tissue sarcoma—an immunoperoxidase study. Am J Pathol 103:384–389, 1981.
41. Brooks JJ: Immunohistochemistry of soft tissue tumors: myoglobin as a tumor marker for rhabdomyosarcoma. Cancer 50:1757–1763, 1982.
42. Tsokos M, Howard R, Costa J: Immunohistochemical study of alveolar and embryonal rhabdomyosarcoma. Lab Invest 48:148–155, 1983.
43. DeJong ASH, van Vark M, Albus-Lutters CE, van Raamsdonk W, Voute PA: Myosin and myoglobin as tumor markers in the diagnosis of rhabdomyosarcoma: a comparative study. Am J Surg Pathol 8:521–528, 1984.
44. Molenaar WM, Oosterhuis JW, Oosterhuis AM, Ramaekers FCS: Mesenchymal and muscle-specific intermediate filaments (vimentin and desmin) in relation to differentiation in childhood rhabdomyosarcomas. Hum Pathol 16:838–843, 1985.
45. Leader M, Colins M, Patel J, Henry K: Desmin: its value as a marker of muscle-derived tumors using a commercial antibody. Virchows Arch [Pathol Anat] 411:345–349, 1987.
46. Eusebi V, Ceccarelli C, Gorza L, Schiaffino S, Bussolati G: Immunocytochemistry of rhabdomyosarcoma: the use of four different markers. Am J Surg Pathol 10:293–299, 1986.
47. Scupham R, Gilbert EF, Wilde J, Wiedrich TA: Immunohistochemical studies of rhabdomyosarcoma. Arch Pathol Lab Med 110:818–821, 1986.
48. Kahn HJ, Yeger H, Kassim O, Jorgensen AO, Maclennan DH, Baumal R, Smith CR, Phillips MJ: Immunohistochemical and electron microscopic assessment of childhood rhabdomyosarcoma. Cancer 51:1897–1903, 1983.
49. Royds JA, Variend S, Timperley WR, Taylor CB: An investigation of beta enolase as a histological marker of rhabdomyosarcoma. J Clin Pathol 37:905–910, 1984.
50. Mukai M, Iri H, Torikata C, Kageyama K, Morikawa Y, Shimizu K: Immunoperoxidase demonstration of a new muscle protein (Z-protein) in myogenic tumors as a diagnostic aid. Am J Pathol 114:164–170, 1984.
51. Bundtzen JL, Norback DH: The ultrastructure of poorly differentiated rhabdomyosarcomas. Hum Pathol 13:301–313, 1982.

52. Mireau GW, Favara BE: Rhabdomyosarcoma in children: ultrastructural study of 31 cases. Cancer 46:2035–2040, 1980.
53. Turc-Carel C, Lizard-Nacol S, Justrabo E, Favrot M, Philip T, Tabone E: Consistent chromosomal translocation in alveolar rhabdomyosarcoma. Cancer Genet Cytogenet 19: 361–362, 1986.
54. Erlandson RA, Woodruff JM: Peripheral nerve sheath tumors: an electron microscopic study of 43 cases. Cancer 49:273–287, 1982.
55. Ducatman BS, Scheithauer BW, Piepgras DG, Reiman HM, Ilstrup DM: Malignant peripheral nerve sheath tumors: a clinicopathologic study of 120 cases. Cancer 57:2006–2021, 1986.
56. Herrera GA, Reimann BEF, Salinas JA: Malignant schwannomas presenting as malignant fibrous histiocytomas. Ultrastruct Pathol 3:253–261, 1982.
57. DiCarlo EF, Woodruff JM, Bansal M, Erlandson RA: The purely epithelioid malignant peripheral nerve sheath tumor. Am J Surg Pathol 10:478–490, 1986.
58. Garrè C: Über sekundar maligne neurome. Beitr Klin Chir 9:465–495, 1892.
59. Ducatman BS, Scheithauer BW: Malignant peripheral nerve sheath tumors with divergent differentiation. Cancer 54:1049–1057, 1984.
60. Masson P, Martin JF: Rhabdomyomes des nerfs. Bull Assoc Fr Etude Cancer 27:751–767, 1938.
61. Woodruff JL, Chernik NL, Smith MC, Millett WB, Foote FW: Peripheral nerve tumors with rhabdomyosarcomatous differentiation (malignant "triton" tumors). Cancer 32:426–439, 1973.
62. Daimaru Y, Hashimoto H, Enjoji M: Malignant "triton" tumors: a clinicopathologic and immunohistochemical study of nine cases. Hum Pathol 15:768–778, 1984.
63. Brooks JJ, Freeman M, Enterline H: Malignant "triton" tumors: natural history and immunohistochemistry of nine new cases with literature review. Cancer 55:2543–2549, 1985.
64. Ushigome S, Takakuwa T, Hyuga M, Tadokoro M, Shinagawa T: Perineurial cell tumor and the significance of the perineurial cells in neurofibroma. Arch Pathol Jpn 36:973–987, 1986.
65. Weidenheim KW, Campbell WG: Perineurial cell tumor: immunocytochemical and ultrastructural characterization—relationship to other peripheral nerve tumors with a review of the literature. Virchows Arch [Pathol Anat] 408:375–383, 1986.
66. Tsuneyoshi M, Enjoji M: Primary malignant peripheral nerve tumors (malignant schwannomas): a clinical and electron microscopic study. Acta Pathol Jpn 29:363–375, 1979.
67. Taxy JB, Battifora H, Trujillo Y, Dorfman HD: Electron microscopy and the diagnosis of malignant schwannoma. Cancer 48:1381–1391, 1981.
68. Chitale AR, Dickersin GR: Electron microscopy in the diagnosis of malignant schwannomas: a report of six cases. Cancer 51:1448–1461, 1983.
69. Arpornchayanon O, Hirota T, Itabashi M, Nakajima T, Fukuma H, Beppu Y, Nishikawa K: Malignant peripheral nerve tumors: a clinicopathological and electron microscopic study. Jpn J Clin Oncol 14:57–74, 1984.
70. Herrera GA, De Moraes HP: Neurogenic sarcoma in patients with neurofibromatosis (von Recklinghausen's disease): light, electron microscopy and immunohistochemistry study. Virchows Arch [Pathol Anat] 403:361–376, 1984.
71. DiMaio SM, Mackay B, Smith JL, Dickersin GR: Neurosarcomatous transformation in malignant melanoma: an ultrastructural study. Cancer 50:2345–2354, 1982.
72. Benson JD, Kraemer BB, Mackay B: Malignant melanoma of soft parts: an ultrastructural study of four cases. Ultrastruct Pathol 8:57–70, 1985.
73. Weiss SW, Langloss JM, Enzinger FM: Value of S100 protein in the diagnosis of soft tissue tumours with particular reference to benign and malignant Schwann cell tumours. Lab Invest 49:299–308, 1983.
74. Daimaru Y, Hashimoto H, Enjoji M: Malignant peripheral nerve sheath tumors (malignant schwannomas): an immunohistochemical study of 29 cases. Am J Surg Pathol 9:434–444, 1985.

75. Matsunou H, Shimoda T, Kakimoto S, Yamashita H, Ishikawa E, Mukai M: Histopathologic and immunohistochemical study of malignant tumors of peripheral nerve sheath (malignant schwannoma). Cancer 56:2269–2279, 1985.

76. Abo T, Balch CH: A differentiation antigen of human NK and K cells identified by a monoclonal antibody (HNK-1). J Immunol 127:1024–1029, 1981.

77. McGarry RC, Helfand SL, Quarles RH, Roder JC: Recognition of myelin-associated glycoprotein by the monoclonal antibody HNK-1. Nature 306:376–378, 1983.

78. Perentes E, Rubinstein LJ: Immunohistochemical recognition of human nerve sheath tumors by anti-Leu 7 (HNK-1) monoclonal antibody. Acta Neuropathol (Berl) 68:319–324, 1985.

79. Swanson PE, Manivel JC, Wick MR: Immunoreactivity for Leu 7 in neurofibrosarcoma and other spindle cell sarcomas of soft tissue. Am J Pathol 126:546–560, 1987.

80. Wick MR, Swanson PE, Scheithauer BW, Manivel JC: Malignant peripheral nerve sheath tumour: an immunohistochemical study of 62 cases. Am J Clin Pathol 87:425–433, 1987.

81. Abenoza P, Manivel C, Swanson PE, Wick MR: Synovial sarcoma: an ultrastructural study, and an immunocytochemical analysis using a combined PAP–ABC procedure. Hum Pathol 17:1107–1115, 1986.

82. Gould VE, Moll R, Moll I, Lee I, Schwechheimer K, Franke WW: The intermediate filament complement of the spectrum of nerve sheath neoplasms. Lab Invest 55:463–474, 1986.

83. Gabbiani G, Kapanci Y, Barrazone P, Franke WW: Immunochemical identification of intermediate-sized filaments in human neoplastic cells: a diagnostic acid for the surgical pathologist. Am J Pathol 104:206–216, 1981.

84. Miettinen M, Lehto V-P, Badley RA, Virtanen I: Expression of intermediate filaments in soft tissue sarcomas. Int J Cancer 30:541–546, 1982.

85. Denk H, Krepler R, Artlieb U, Gabbiani G, Rungger-Brandle E, Leoncini P, Franke WW: Proteins of intermediate filaments: an immunohistochemical and biochemical approach to the classification of soft tissue tumors. Am J Pathol 110:193–208, 1983.

86. Osborn M, Altmannsberger M, Debus E, Weber K: Differentiation of the major human tumor groups using conventional and monoclonal antibodies specific for individual intermediate filament proteins. Ann NY Acad Sci 455:649–668, 1985.

87. Hashimoto H, Daimaru Y, Tsuneyoshi M, Enjoji M: Leiomyosarcoma of the external soft tissues: a clinicopathologic, immunohistochemical, and electron microscopic study. Cancer 57:2077–2088, 1986.

88. Ryan GB, Cliff WJ, Gabbiani G, Irle C, Montandou D, Statkov PR, Majno G: Myofibroblasts in human granulation tissue. Hum Pathol 5:55–67, 1974.

89. Rosai J, Sumner H, Kostianowsky M, Perez-Mesa C: Angiosarcoma of the skin: a clinicopathologic and fine structural study. Hum Pathol 7:83–109, 1976.

90. Maddox J, Evans H: Angiosarcoma of the skin and soft tissue: a study of 44 cases. Cancer 48:1907–1921, 1981.

91. Donnell R, Kay S, Rosen P, Braun D, Lieberman P, Kinne D, Kaufman R: Angiosarcoma and other vascular tumors of the breast: pathologic analysis as a guide to prognosis. Am J Surg Pathol 5:629–642, 1981.

92. Hoyer LW, de los Santos RP, Hoyer IR: Antihemophilic factor antigen: localisation in endothelial cells by immunofluorescence microscopy. J Clin Invest 52:2737–2744, 1973.

93. Mukai K, Rosai J, Burgdorf WHC: Localisation of factor VIII-related antigen in vascular endothelial cells using an immunoperoxidase method. Am J Surg Pathol 4:273–276, 1980.

94. Burgdorf WHC, Mukai K, Rosai J: Immunohistochemical identification of factor VIII-related antigen in endothelial cells of cutaneous lesions of alleged vascular nature. Am J Clin Pathol 75:167–171, 1981.

95. Miettinen M, Holthofer H, Lehto V-P, Miettinen A, Virtanen I: Ulex europaeus 1 lectin as a marker for tumours derived from endothelial cells. Am J Clin Pathol 79:32–36, 1983.

96. Ordonez NG, Batsakis JG: Comparison of Ulex europaeus 1 lectin with factor VIII-related antigen in vascular lesions. Arch Pathol Lab Med 108:129–132, 1984.

97. Weiss SW, Enzinger FM: Epithelioid hemangioendothelioma: a vascular tumor often

mistaken for a carcinoma. Cancer 50:970–981, 1982.

98. Ishak KG, Sesterhenn IA, Goodman ZD, Rabin L, Stromeyer FW: Epithelioid hemangio-endothelioma of the liver: a clinicopathologic and follow-up study of 32 cases. Hum Pathol 15:839–852, 1984.
99. Ackerman AB: Subtle clues to the diagnosis by conventional microscopy: the patch stage of Kaposi's sarcoma. Am J Dermatopathol 1:165–172, 1979.
100. Rutgers J, Wieczorek R, Bonetti F, Kaplan K, Posnett D, Friedman-Klein A, Knowles D: The expression of endothelial cell surface antigens by AIDS-associated Kaposi's sarcoma: evidence for a vascular endothelial cell origin. Am J Pathol 122:493–499, 1986.
101. Brooks JJ: Kaposi's sarcoma: a reversible hyperplasia. Lancet 2:1309–1311, 1986.
102. Real FX, Krown SE: Spontaneous regression of Kaposi's sarcoma in patients with AIDS. N Engl J Med 313:1659, 1985.
103. Enzinger FM, Smith BH: Haemangiopericytoma: analysis of 106 cases. Hum Pathol 7:61–82, 1976.
104. Hoffman MA, Dickersin GR: Malignant fibrous histiocytoma: an ultrastructural study of eleven cases. Hum Pathol 14:913–922, 1983.
105. Miettinen M, Lehto VP, Virtanen I: Monophasic synovial sarcoma of spindle cell type: epithelial differentiation as revealed by ultrastructural features, content of prekeratin and binding of peanut agglutinin. Virchows Arch [Cell Pathol] 44:187–199, 1983.
106. Corson JM, Weiss LM, Banks-Schlegel SP, Pinkus GS: Keratin proteins and carcino-embryonic antigen in synovial sarcomas: an immunohistochemical study of 24 cases. Hum Pathol 15:615–621, 1984.
107. Fisher C: Synovial sarcoma: ultrastructural and immunohistochemical features of epithelial differentiation in monophasic and biphasic tumours. Hum Pathol 17:996–1008, 1986.
108. Michelson MR, Brown GA, Maynard JA, Cooper RR, Bonfiglio M: Synovial sarcoma: an electron microscopic study of monophasic and biphasic forms. Cancer 45:2109–2118, 1980.
109. Krall RA, Kostianovsky M, Patchefsky AS: Synovial sarcoma: a clinical, pathological and ultrastructural study of 26 cases supporting the recognition of a monophasic variant. Am J Surg Pathol 5:137–151, 1981.
110. Turc-Carel C, Dal Cin P, Rao U, Karakousis C, Sandberg AA: Translocation X:18 in synovial sarcoma. Cancer Genet Cytogenet 23:93–94, 1986.
111. Smith S, Reeves BR, Wong L, Fisher C: A consistent chromosome translocation in synovial sarcoma. Cancer Genet Cytogenet 26:179–180, 1987.
112. Miettinen M, Virtanen I: Synovial sarcoma: a misnomer. Am J Pathol 117:18–25, 1984.
113. Soule EH: Synovial sarcoma. Am J Surg Pathol 10:78–82, 1986.
114. Evans H: A study of 23 biphasic and 17 probable monophasic examples. Pathol Annu 15:309–331, 1980.
115. Cagle LA, Mirra JM, Storm K, Roe JD, Eilber FR: Histologic features relating to prognosis in synovial sarcoma. Cancer 59:1810–1814, 1987.
116. Varela-Duran J, Enzinger FM: Calcifying synovial sarcoma. Cancer 50:345–352, 1982.
117. Enzinger F: Epithelioid sarcoma: a sarcoma simulating a granuloma or a carcinoma. Cancer 26:1029–1041, 1970.
118. Chase DR, Enzinger FM: Epithelioid sarcoma: diagnosis, prognostic indicators, and treatment. Am J Surg Pathol 9:241–263, 1985.
119. Chase DR, Weiss SW, Enzinger FM, Langloss JM: Keratin in epithelioid sarcoma: an immunohistochemical study. Am J Surg Pathol 8:435–441, 1984.
120. Mukai M, Torikata C, Iri H, Hanaoka H, Kawai T, Yakumaru K, Shimoda T, Mikata A, Kageyama K: Cellular differentiation of epithelioid sarcoma: an electron-microscopic, enzyme-histochemical, and immunohistochemical study. Am J Pathol 119:44–56, 1985.
121. Wick MR, Manivel JC: Epithelioid sarcoma and isolated necrobiotic granuloma: a comparative immunocytochemical study. J Cutan Pathol 13:253–260, 1986.
122. Fisher C: Epithelioid sarcoma: the spectrum of ultrastructural differentiation in seven immunohistochemically defined cases. Hum Pathol 19:265–275, 1988.
123. Sloane JP, Ormerod MG: Distribution of epithelial membrane antigen in normal and

neoplastic tissues and its value in diagnostic tumor pathology. Cancer 47:1786–1795, 1981.

124. Reeves BR, Fisher C, Smith S, Courtenay D, Robertson D: Ultrastructural, immunocyto-chemical and cytogenetic characterisation of a human epithelioid sarcoma cell line (RM-HS1). J Natl Cancer Inst 78:7–18, 1987.

125. Enzinger FM: Clear cell sarcoma of tendons and aponeuroses: an analysis of 21 cases. Cancer 18:1163–1174, 1965.

126. Pavlidis N, Fisher C, Wiltshaw E: Clear cell sarcoma of tendons and aponeuroses: a clinico-pathologic study. Cancer 54:1412–1417, 1984.

127. Hajdu SI, Shiu MH, Fortner JG: Tendosynovial sarcoma: a clinicopathological study of 136 cases. Cancer 39:1201–1217, 1977.

128. Kindblom L-G, Lodding P, Angervall L: Clear cell sarcoma of tendons and aponeuroses: an immunohistochemical and electron microscopic analysis indicating neural crest origin. Virchows Arch [Pathol Anat] 401:109–128, 1983.

129. Chung EB, Enzinger FM: Malignant melanoma of soft parts: a reassessment of clear cell sarcoma. Am J Surg Pathol 7:405–413, 1983.

130. Mukai M, Torikata C, Iri H, Mikata A, Kawai T, Hanaoka H, Yakumaru K, Kageyama K: Histogenesis of clear cell sarcoma of tendons and aponeuroses: an electron microscopic, biochemical, enzyme histochemical, and immunohistochemical study. Am J Pathol 114: 264–272, 1984.

131. Benson JD, ..raemer BB, Mackay B: Malignant melanoma of soft parts: an ultrastructural study of four cases. Ultrastruct Pathol 8:57–70, 1985.

132. Christopherson WM, Foote FW, Stewart FW: Alveolar soft-part sarcomas: structurally characteristic tumors of uncertain histogenesis. Cancer 5:100–111, 1952.

133. De Schryver-Kecskemeti K, Kraus FT, Engleman W, Lacy PE: Alveolar soft-part sarcoma: a malignant angioreninoma—histochemical, immunocytochemical, and electron-micro-scopic study of four cases. Am J Surg Pathol 6:5–18, 1982.

134. Mukai M, Torikata C, Iri H, Mikata A, Sakamoto T, Hanaoka H, Shinohara C, Baba N, Kanaya K, Kageyama K: Alveolar soft part sarcoma: an elaboration of a three-dimensional configuration of the crystalloids by digital image processing. Am J Pathol 116:398–406, 1984.

135. Mathew T: Evidence supporting neural crest origin of an alveolar soft part sarcoma: an ultrastructural study. Cancer 50:507–514, 1982.

136. Fisher ER, Reidbord H: Electron microscopic evidence suggesting the myogenous deriva-tion of the so-called alveolar soft part sarcoma. Cancer 27:150–159, 1971.

137. Mukai M, Torikata C, Iri H, Mikata A, Hanaoka H, Kato K, Kageyama K: Histogenesis of alveolar soft part sarcoma: an immunohistochemical and biochemical study. Am J Surg Pathol 10:212–218, 1986.

138. Auerbach HE, Brooks JJ: Alveolar soft part sarcoma: a clinicopathologic and immuno-histochemical study. Cancer 60:66–73, 1987.

139. Lieberman PH, Foote FW, Stewart FW, Berg JW: Alveolar soft-part sarcoma. JAMA 198:1047–1051, 1966.

140. Evans HL: Alveolar soft part sarcoma: a study of 13 typical examples and one with a histo-logically atypical component. Cancer 55:912–917, 1985.

141. Nakamura Y, Becker LE, Marks A: S-100 protein in tumors of cartilage and bone: an immunohistochemical study. Cancer 52:1820–1824, 1983.

142. Miettinen M: Chordoma: antibodies to epithelial membrane antigen and carcinoembryonic antigen in differential diagnosis. Arch Pathol Lab Med 108:891–892, 1984.

143. Salisbury JR, Isaacson PG: Demonstration of cytokeratins and an epithelial membrane antigen in chordomas and human fetal notochord. Am J Surg Pathol 9:791–797, 1985.

144. Abenoza P, Sibley RK: Chordoma: an immunohistologic study. Hum Pathol 17:744–747, 1986.

145. Povysil C, Matejovsky Z: A comparative ultrastructural study of chondrosarcoma, chordoid sarcoma, chordoma, and chordoma periphericum. Pathol Res Pract 179:546–559, 1985.

146. Monda L, Wick MR: S100 protein immunostaining in the differential diagnosis of chondro-

blastoma. Hum Pathol 16:287–293, 1985.

147. Chung EB, Enzinger FM: Extraskeletal osteosarcoma. Cancer 60:1132–1142, 1987.

148. Angervall L, Enzinger FM: Extraskeletal neoplasm resembling Ewing's sarcoma. Cancer 36:240–251, 1975.

149. Soule EH, Newton W, Moon TE, Tefft M: Extraskeletal Ewing's sarcoma: a preliminary review of 26 cases encountered in the Intergroup Rhabdomyosarcoma Study. Cancer 42: 259–264, 1978.

150. Stuart-Harris R, Wills EJ, Philips J, Langlands AO, Fox RM, Tattersall MHN: Extraskeletal Ewing's sarcoma: a clinical, morphological and ultrastructural analysis of five cases with a review of the literature. Eur J Cancer Clin Oncol 22:393–400, 1986.

151. Navas-Palacios JJ, Aparicio-Duque R, Valdes MD: On the histogenesis of Ewing's sarcoma: an ultrastructural, immunohistochemical and cytochemical study. Cancer 53:1882–1901, 1984.

152. Moll R, Lee I, Gould VE, Berndt R, Roessner A, Franke WW: Immunocytochemical analysis of Ewing's tumors: patterns of expression of intermediate filaments and desmosomal proteins indicate cell type heterogeneity and pluripotential differentiation. Am J Pathol 127:288–304, 1987.

153. Miettinen M, Lehto V-P, Virtanen I: Histogenesis of Ewing's sarcoma: an evaluation of intermediate filaments and endothelial cell markers. Virchows Arch [Cell Pathol] 41: 277–284, 1982.

154. Aurias A, Rimbaut C, Buffe D, Dubousset J, Mazabraud A: Chromosomal translocations in Ewing's sarcoma. N Engl J Med 309–496–497, 1983.

155. Turc-Carel C, Philip I, Berger M-P, Philip T, Lenoir GM: Chromosomal translocations in Ewing's sarcoma. N Engl J Med 309:497–498, 1983.

156. Maletz N, McMorrow LE, Greco MA, Wolman SR: Ewing's sarcoma: pathology, tissue culture and cytogenetics. Cancer 58:252–257, 1986.

157. Suit HD, Mankin HJ, Schiller AL, Wood WC, Tepper JE: Staging systems for sarcoma of soft tissue and sarcoma of bone. Cancer Treat Symp 3:29–36, 1985.

158. Tetu B, Hunt A, McCaughey WTE, Lagace R: Evaluation des divergences d'opinion sur le diagnostic histopatholoqique des tumeurs des tissues mous. Ann Pathol 4:267–271, 1984.

159. Coindre JM, Trojani M, Contesso G, David M, Rouesse J, Buji NB, Bodaert A, De Mascarel I, De Mascarel A, Goussot J-F: Reproducibility of a histopathologic grading system for adult soft tissue sarcoma. Cancer 58:306–309, 1986.

160. Myhre-Jensen O, Kaae S, Madsen EH, Sneppen O: Histopathological grading in soft tissue tumours: relation to survival in 261 surgically treated patients. Acta Pathol Microbiol Scand [A] 91:145–150, 1983.

161. De Stefani E, Deneo-Pellegrini H, Carzoglio J, Cendan ME, Vassalo A, Coppola J, Olivera L, Viola A: Sarcomes des tissus mous: facteurs histologiques de prognostic. Bull Cancer 69:443–450, 1982.

162. Trojani M, Contesso G, Coindre JM, Rouesse J, Bui NB, De Mascarel A, Goussot JF, David M, Bonichon F, Lagarde C: Soft-tissue sarcomas of adults: study of pathologic prognostic variables and definition of a histopathological grading system. Int J Cancer 33: 37–42, 1984.

163. Markhede G, Angervall L, Stener B: A multivariate analysis of the prognosis after surgical treatment of malignant soft-tissue tumors. Cancer 49:1721–1733, 1982.

164. Collin C, Godbold J, Hajdu S, Brennan M: Localized extremity soft tissue sarcoma: an analysis of factors affecting survival. J Clinc Oncol 5:601–612, 1987.

165. Heise HW, Myers MH, Russell WO, Suit HD, Enzinger FM, Edmonson JH, Cohen J, Martin RG, Miller WT, Hajdu SI: Recurrence-free survival time for surgically-treated soft tissue sarcoma patients. Cancer 57:172–177, 1986.

166. Rydholm A, Berg NO, Gullberg BO, Thorngren KG, Persson BM: Epidemiology of soft-tissue sarcoma in the locomotor system. Acta Pathol Microbiol Scand [A] 92:363–374, 1984.

2. Diagnostic imaging

Richard P. Golding, Thea E.G. van Zanten, and Jaap Valk

In growth, soft tissue sarcomas displace the contents and later the boundaries of the anatomical space in which they arise. Linear extension does occur, however, along neurovascular bundles. Blood-borne spread occurs to the lungs. Less often or later spread to the liver, bones, and brain may take place. Involvement of lymph nodes is said to occur infrequently [1, 2] and is probably related to tumor size and an unfavorable prognosis. Within the group of childhood rhabdomyosarcomas, the incidence of lymph node involvement is variable, being highest for prostatic, genitourinary, and paratesticular sites and very low for head, neck, and truncal sites [3]. In general, the incidence of lymph node metastases from soft tissue sarcomas is usually low, certainly in comparison to those for the commonly occurring carcinomas [4].

Although surgical resection is still the mainstay of treatment, local recurrence is a problem of particular importance after local and wide resection and even after amputation [5]. Surgery has also been recommended in the treatment of pulmonary metastases where repeated resections can achieve prolonged survival [6]. Although the great majority of pulmonary metastases are peripherally located and thus amenable to wedge resection, endobronchial metastases have been described [7]. Similarly although the presentation of soft tissue sarcomas is straightforward, as a rarity a paraneoplastic syndrome involving hypoglycemia, hyperglycemia, anemia, or hypercalcemia without skeletal metastases may be encountered [8].

The ability of imaging methods to provide information on the different states of soft tissue sarcomas has been the subject of previous reviews, but a continuing addition of newer methods of imaging has entailed reappraisals [9, 10]. If investment in medical imaging technology continues, we will see not only advances in existing techniques, but completely new instruments.

Imaging methods

Plain films and xeroradiography

Although these lack almost as much sensitivity as they do specificity, plain films are frequently requested as the first imaging examination probably

Pinedo, H.M., Verweij, J., eds. TREATMENT OF SOFT TISSUE SARCOMAS.

because the diagnosis of a soft tissue sarcoma has not been seriously entertained. Inasmuch as displacement of fascial planes, or the presence of calcifications or low-density elements, may endorse the results of palpation or confirm a clinical suspicion, plain films have worth. However, the most important contribution of plain radiography is likely to be the demonstration of involvement of adjacent skeletal structures when this exists. There is anecdotal evidence that malignant change in a lipoma has been detected as an increase in density in the low-density fatty tissue subsequent to an increase in stromal elements. Xeroradiography can show calcific and fatty structures better than conventional radiographs. It has no other particular advantages, however. One report examining a variety of malignant and benign soft tissue lesions found that xeroradiography detected periosteal resections better than ultrasound or computed tomography, but that plain radiographs reliably though less impressively detected these same changes [11].

Tomography

This technique is still of use in examining the ear, the paranasal sinuses, and the upper airways. Doubtful bony lesions seen on plain films may also be much more clearly shown on tomograms. In general, however, tomography has been giving way to computer tomography (CT) in almost every area. In the thorax, it now no longer seems appropriate to subject patients to tomography especially for staging and follow-up of malignant neoplasms when CT is available. The latter will detect more pulmonary nodules as well as visualizing the mediastinum, pleura, chest wall, and skeleton in one session.

Angiography and lymphangiography

Angiography is still a useful procedure. However, there has been a definite shift in the application of this technique. Whereas formerly it was primarily used as a diagnostic method firstly to establish a diagnosis of malignancy and secondly to establish the extent of the lesion, it is now used in its diagnostic capacity for vascular mapping and in its therapeutic capacity for various embolization procedures and for the placement of catheters for intra-arterial chemotherapy.

With regard to angiography as a diagnostic method, an interesting development has been the use of intra-arterial digital subtraction angiography (DSA). In one study used to evaluate 36 patients with limb tumors, 14 of which were soft tissue sarcomas, major arteries both normal and abnormal and feeding arteries were equally well shown by both conventional arteriography and intra-arterial DSA [12]. Extremely small vessels tended to be beyond the resolution of a 512×512 matrix. However, large but faint shadows such as tumor stains or draining veins were just as clearly visible on the electronically subtracted images as on the radiographs. The major advantage was the lack of discomfort suffered by the patients during the injection of a dilute contrast material (73 mg iodine/ml). The new procedure was also cheaper and somewhat quicker.

Lymphangiography should in theory have an advantage over CT in that it can detect filling defects due to tumor deposits in normal-sized nodes and is not dependent on enlargement of nodes as is CT for a diagnosis of lymphadenopathy. In addition, CT has difficulty in detecting enlargement in the vertical axis on transverse cuts. Even in the transverse plane, there is no universal agreement as to what should be accepted as an enlarged transverse diameter without, on the one hand, reaping too many false positives while retaining a high percentage of the true negatives or, on the other hand, reversing this with too many false negatives and too few true positives when the chosen nodal diameters are too small or too big, respectively. This perennial problem is bound up with the fact that normal lymph nodes show a range of sizes, and lymph node enlargement can be due to inflammation rather than invasion. In practice, however, the limited applications of lymphangiography to the various lymph node chains in the body and frequent failure of extensively involved nodes to take up contrast give CT a definite advantage over lymphangiography.

Isotopes

The uses of isotope scanning include the detection of the primary lesion, including recurrence after resection, involvement of adjacent bones, and the detection of distant metastases. Since certain isotope scanning agents localize in soft tissue sarcomas, the first objective can be met but is, in practice, of little value since small tumors are not reliably detected. With regard to the involvement of adjacent bone, a study of 60 patients with soft tissue sarcomas by using technetium-99m-labeled pyrophosphate or methylene diphosphonate reported a 92% accuracy in determining the presence or absence of bone involvement [13]. In 54 patients, however, this information endorsed that available from other sources and in only one case provided information not otherwise available. A later study from the same center [14] compared bone scintigraphy and CT. Although this study comprised only 17 patients selected from 139, none of these had been biopsied or irradiated before the imaging studies, none had plain film evidence of bone erosion or periosteal reaction, and all had optimal surgical and radiological documentation. Using technetium-99m-labeled ethylene or methylene diphosphonate, scintigrams were obtained using multiple projections when these were necessary to display tumor activity separate from adjacent bone activity. When no normal intervening tissue could be demonstrated, bone involvement was considered to be present. There were no false-negative or false-positive scintigrams. Three computed tomograms incorrectly diagnosed bone involvement. The anatomical definition of bone involvement was the extension of either the tumor or the surrounding reactive edematous tissue to the periosteum or cortical bone, with or without direct invasion of these structures in the case of tumor.

Using gallium-67-labeled citrate, activity has been shown in the primary tumor in 41 of 48 patients known to have a soft tissue sarcoma of the extremity at the time of imaging [15]. Seven other patients with histological evidence of residual tumor had negative gallium scans. Interestingly six patients with positive scans also had evidence of nonpulmonary metastatic disease (mostly lymphadenopathy) that was later supported by other data.

The mechanism by which the scanning agents mentioned above localize in tumor tissue is not entirely clear. Preliminary work on a more specific approach has recently been reported by Hoefnagel et al. [16], who used antibody fragments directed against myosin, which is known to be present in rhabdomyosarcoma cells. Early results were encouraging in detecting primary, recurrent, and metastatic tumor.

Ultrasound

A recent report described the use of ultrasound as a screening study in the evaluation of soft tissue masses. All patients had a palpable mass or palpably altered tissue consistency, no abnormalities on plain radiographs, no biopsy procedure prior to ultrasonography, and all had adequate ultrasonographic and histological data available for review [17]. Of these 50 patients, 14 had a malignant lesion which in each case was sonographically discrete and well defined and, in one case, cystic. Those with benign lesions had either discrete or else ill-defined lesions that were not easily distinguishable from surrounding tissues; 13 of these benign lesions were cystic although this was sonographically apparent in only seven cases. The authors point out that there appeared to be a correlation between histologic and ultrasonographic patterns inasmuch as the discrete lesions, with a uniformly decreased echogenicity in comparison to surrounding tissues, had a high cell-to-matrix ratio whether they were benign or malignant. As already indicated, all ill-defined lesions (with a low cell-to-matrix index similar to that of surrounding tissue) encountered in the study were benign.

The patients in the study cited above are not representative of patients with soft tissue abnormalities seeking medical advice for the first time. All had been referred to a teaching hospital presumably because of clinical suspicion and indeed a quarter had a soft tissue malignancy. It may therefore be premature to accept their findings as valid for large-scale screening. The authors, however, are surely right to advocate ultrasound as the first imaging examination instead of plain radiographs where physical examination suggests a soft tissue abnormality.

Computed tomography

As first- and second-generation scanners were replaced by third- and fourth-generation scanners, the enthusiasm of early reports of the usefulness of the preoperative imaging of the location and extension of soft tissue tumors by computer tomography (CT) [18–20] was amply confirmed by later reports [21–23]. However, it became clear that although excellent depiction of the tumor and the anatomical compartment in which it was located was often possible, in a number of cases depiction of the margins of the tumor even with intravenous contrast enhancement was unreliable as ascertained at subsequent surgery. Early reports had already indicated that the hope that CT might, on the basis of its superb contrast sensitivity and spatial resolution, be able to attempt tissue characterization was, in the main, unfounded. Lipomas could often be identified, but poorly differentiated liposarcomas could not be confidently distinguished from other neoplasms that might contain areas of low density due to cystic or necrotic changes. Well-differentiated liposarcomas have been confused with lipomas. It also became apparent that positive CT diagnoses such as vascular encasement, regional lymphadenopathy, or local bone destruction were more likely to be confirmed at operation than were CT diagnoses excluding such pathology. Problems also arose with the main seeding ground for metastases, the lung parenchyma, for, although CT showed more nodules than could be seen on chest radiographs or tomograms, not all of these nodules proved to be metastases at operation. Finally, CT has been shown to have limited value following excisional biopsy [24]. In this study, an attempt was made to identify those patients with residual macroscopic tumor following marginal excision since these patients would require additional measures to prevent local recurrence and to distinguish this group from those who had only postoperative reactive changes where the presumed presence of microscopic deposits would be an indication for local radiotherapy. CT was not reliable in detecting malignancy when no palpable mass was present, nor when a palpable mass was present was CT reliable in distinguishing between malignancy and postoperative changes.

In conclusion, it may be stated that CT depicts soft tissue sarcomas and surrounding structures in detail, giving information considered to be superior to that provided by ultrasound and angiography. As a diagnostic method, however, for staging and follow-up, it has important limitations that four generations of scanners have not eliminated. Its great strength lies in the fact that, at the time of writing, it is the only imaging technique that is in general use that can provide anatomically detailed images of virtually all systems. In our institution, it is the preferred method of screening for pulmonary, cerebral, and hepatic metastases in addition to preoperative assessment of the primary neoplasm.

Magnetic resonance: imaging and spectroscopy

The early course of magnetic resonance (MR) was to some extent a recapitulation of the development of CT. MR's first and most successful application was in the central nervous system. Early hopes that MR might provide tissue characterization, at least the distinction between benign and malignant lesions, have not as yet been realized.

When imaging soft tissue tumors, both T1 and T2 weighted sequences are recommended for the best delineation of the lesion, but these sequences do not allow a distinction between benign and malignant lesions [25]. One report has claimed to distinguish lipomas from liposarcomas on the basis of calculations of T1 and T2 relaxation times [26]. However, the number of liposarcomas was small (two) and their differentiation grade was not stated. On the other hand, the signal emanating from the tissues adjacent to a soft tissue malignancy has been found to be increased [27]. In seven of nine cases of soft tissue sarcomas in which this was observed, either edema or tumor invasion of the adjacent muscle tissue was found on histology. Benign soft tissue tumors did not show this sign but inflammatory lesions did. Comparisons between CT and MR in the evaluation of both primary soft tissue tumors and bone tumors with soft tissue extension have generally found the two techniques to be at least comparable, with MR tending to be superior in some respects, particularly with regard to lesion extension within the soft tissues and bone marrow [28–30]. Similar results have also been found in children [31].

As an imaging method, MR is much more complex than CT, both for the manufacturer and the user. Optimal magnetic field strengths and pulse sequences have yet to be determined. Some attempts have already been made to establish the MR factors likely to produce the best results. Both the visibility and the apparent size of lesions were found to vary with the imaging technique employed [32].

Apart from MR clinical imaging, a certain amount of in vitro work has also been reported. Using a formula based on combinations of T1 and T2 values of surgical specimens examined in a hydrogen nuclear MR spectrometer, one report describes the correct differentiation between benign and malignant lesions in all 27 soft tissue specimens examined [33]. More recent work has used proton MR spectroscopy to examine small tumor samples to determine T2 relaxation times characteristic of cells with metastatic potential [34]. Phosphorus (^{31}P) MR spectra have also been obtained in vivo from superficial tumors by using surface coils. All tumors examined had a raised intracellular pH. Other abnormalities were observed, but as yet no coherent pattern has emerged [35].

Imaging affected areas

Head and neck

A review of 188 cases of soft tissue sarcomas of the head and neck in adults and adolescents found a fairly even distribution of various sarcomas between different anatomical sites [36]. Those sites affected in decreasing order were neck, 23%; face, 20%; sinonasal cavity, 19%; scalp, 18%; upper aerodigestive tract, 11%; and salivary glands and miscellaneous sites, 5% and 4%, respectively. The authors found CT to be valuable both in preoperative staging and

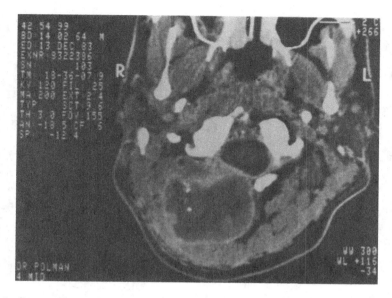

Figure 1. Computed tomographic scan of a paravertebral synovial sarcoma showing ring enhancement of the pseudocapsule. Reproduced from Treu et al. [73], with permission of Raven Press.

in assessing therapeutic response. Soft tissue sarcomas in the head and neck region, as elsewhere in the body, may be surrounded by a pseudocapsule of compressed tissue with a reactive inflammatory zone that may also contain malignant cells. It is this zone that may show ring enhancement following intravenous contrast, as is shown in Fig. 1. This was a case of a paravertebral synovial sarcoma. Other reports concerning synovial sarcomas in the head and neck are less specific about radiological diagnosis [37, 38] although, in a case involving the temporomandibular joint, CT was found to be helpful [39]. Reports dealing with sarcomas of the larynx and nasopharynx indicate the importance of determining local extent of the tumor since recurrence is a major hazard and local lymph node metastases are less of a danger [40–43]. Figure 2 demonstrates the usefulness of MR in determining local extent including, in this case, intracranial extension. One report dealing with soft part sarcoma of the orbit mentions the value of ultrasound although, in this case, both CT and orbital venography were also considered to be of value [44].

Thorax and breast

Soft tissue sarcomas arising in the hollow organs of the mediastinum can be detected by luminal opacification with the appropriate contrast study. However CT of the thorax will provide a more global view and, in addition, simultaneously examine the lungs for metastatic disease. Tumors arising in the mediastinum or chest wall should always be examined by CT. MR is an ac-

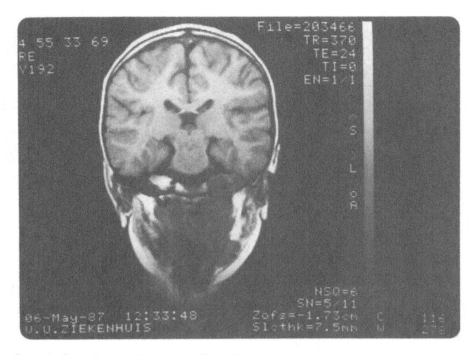

Figure 2. Coronal magnetic resonance illustrating intracranial extension of a nasopharyngeal rhabdomyosarcoma.

ceptable alternative for the primary location, but is, at the time of writing, decidedly inferior to CT for imaging lung parenchyma.

Sarcomas of the breast may occur following previous radiotherapy for carcinoma [45]. Although fibrosarcoma and malignant fibrous histiocytoma are the commonest types, angiosarcoma occurs more commonly in the breast than elsewhere in the body [46]. Mammography may adequately visualize the lesions although deep seated tumors such as many angiosarcomas [47] may be better imaged by xeromammography, which shows not only the retromammary space but also the ribs and pleural region. Where invasion of the chest wall is suspected, CT has been employed [45]. Axillary lymphadenopathy was not found in previous studies [46–48].

Retroperitoneum and intraperitoneal organs

Retroperitoneal soft tissue sarcomas usually present with abdominal or flank pain, weight loss, and a palpable mass [49]. In cases of malignant fibrous histiocytoma in the retroperitoneum or abdomen, features at presentation have also included abdominal distension, varicocele, hernia, fatigue [1], obstructive jaundice [50], inferior vena caval obstruction [51], and nonfunctioning kidney on intravenous urography [52]. Soft tissue sarcomas arising from

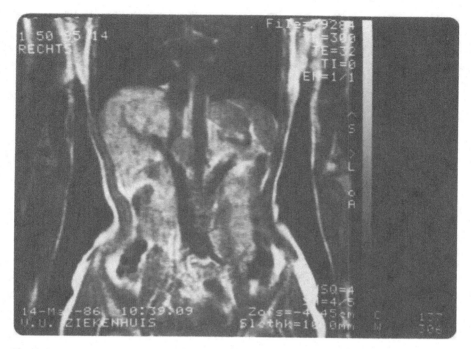

Figure 3. Coronal magnetic resonance illustrating a recurrent leiomyosarcoma of the inferior vena cava confirmed at operation. Reproduced from van Zanten et al. [74], with permission of Raven Press.

retroperitoneal structures may present with more specific features indicating their site of origin. Leiomyosarcomas of the inferior vena cava, for instance, may present with lower-limb edema or the nephrotic or Budd-Chiari syndromes. These tumors may therefore be detected at an earlier stage (see Fig. 3) whereas most primary retroperitoneal sarcomas are found to be very extensive at first operation (see Fig. 4). One-third of cases of hemangiosarcoma of the spleen present with splenic rupture [53]. This diversity of presentation coupled with almost universally limited experience with these rare tumors means that the diagnosis is arrived at indirectly both clinically and radiologically. When a palpable mass is encountered, ultrasound is the easiest means of locating it, but CT or MR is the best means of defining its extent. The use of preoperative CT has been advocated in reports in the surgical literature emphasizing the importance of radical surgery as the most effective therapy [54].

A review of sarcomas of the stomach [55] established leiomyosarcoma as the most commonly occurring type (95%), the fundus and body as the predominant sites, and adverse prognostic factors to be tumor diameter of 8 cm or more and extension to the serosal surface. Metastatic disease to the liver and regional lymph nodes as well as extragastric extension of tumor to neighboring organs were common. As might be expected from this description, CT

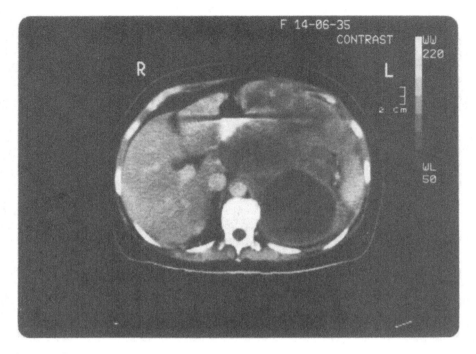

Figure 4. Computer tomographic scan of a retroperitoneal liposarcoma demonstrating fatty and dense stromal elements, some surrounded by highly vascularized areas showing ring enhancement after bolus contrast injection.

is the most appropriate form of imaging for these tumors although some case studies report the successful use of ultrasound [56]. We have been impressed by the extent to which extraluminal growth of gut neoplasms in general as shown on CT can occur without clinical evidence of obstruction [57].

Leiomyosarcomas of the large bowel have more or less the same incidence as occurs in the small intestine, and a review of the latter [58] indicates a propensity for exoenteric growth and distant metastasis before lymph node involvement. Mesenteric arteriography was useful, but barium studies were insensitive, although it is not stated whether the small bowel enema technique was used. When this technique is employed, excellent delineation of tumorous masses can be achieved although the exact extraluminal extent still requires another imaging technique such as CT (see Fig. 5).

Limbs

A review of soft tissue sarcomas of the distal extremities [59] listed the following histologic types in order of decreasing frequency: synovial cell, fibrosarcoma, liposarcoma, and rhabdomyosarcoma. When the proximal extremities are included, there would probably be a shift toward liposarcoma and malignant fibrous histiocytoma [1, 60]. A review of musculoskeletal liposarcomas

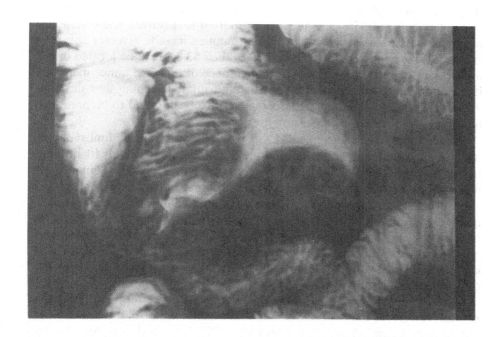

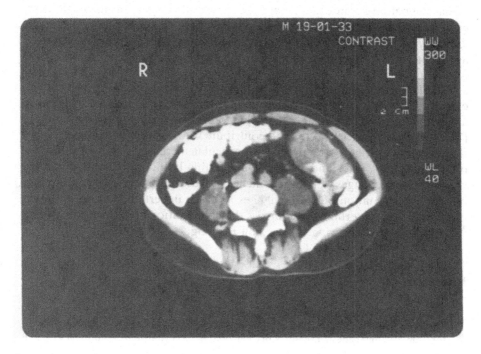

Figure 5A and B. Small bowel enema and computer tomography excellently delineate the mucosal and extraluminal extension of this synovial sarcoma metastasized from the knee.

[60] found slightly more than half of these in the proximal lower extremity. A similar figure of 65% has also been reported [61]. Other less commonly occurring soft tissue sarcomas in the extremities include alveolar soft-part sarcoma. Lieberman et al. [62] found 50 of their 53 cases to be located in the limbs. An isolated report of the CT appearance of this rare tumor mentions its strongly enhancing appearance with both dilated feeding and draining vessels [63]. Extraskeletal osteosarcoma has also been found to be predominantly (67%) located in the extremities [64].

Early reports of CT diagnosis of soft tissue sarcomas of the limbs all emphasize its value in clearly visualizing the lesion and in accurately identifying the anatomical compartment in which it has arisen [65–67]. This is important when either an intracompartmental or extracompartmental en bloc resection is being considered as described by Enneking et al. [68]. More recent reports, however, have been more cautious and the "pernicious growth characteristics of sarcomas, which send out fingerlike projections along fascial planes and muscle bundles" [36] has seeped into the awareness of both radiologists and clinicians alike. Two reports of CT of childhood synovial sarcomas stress the difficulty in accurately defining tumor margins [69, 70].

When compared with CT, MR has been found to be better in outlining the size and extent of tumors and their relationship to major blood vessels, but not so good in detecting bone destruction [71]. This study employed a 0.5 Tesla magnet and spin echo T1 and T2 weighted images. In our institution, using very similar technical factors, we have not been aware of any particular difficulty in detecting erosion of bone. Soft tissue calcifications may not be apparent on MR, but our recent experience with gradient echoes in this field is encouraging.

Finally, it seems appropriate to mention a pilot study using surface coils to obtain ^{31}P spectra from extremity bone tumors since this may be even more applicable to some soft tissue tumors due to their proximity to the skin surface [72]. Overlying muscles do tend to contribute to the sampling volume. Nonetheless some changes were noted, in particular increased levels of phosphodiester and monoester and also ATP suggesting both aerobic and anaerobic regions. Other changes were noted, including a decrease in phosphocreatinine, but the interpretation of these changes is as yet uncertain. Future improvements will almost certainly encompass the combination of surface coil ^{1}H and ^{31}P spectroscopy following surface coil imaging.

References

1. Weiss SW, Enzinger FM: Malignant fibrous histiocytoma. Cancer 41:2250–2266, 1978.
2. Lawrence W Jr, Hays DM, Heyn R, Tefft M, Crist W, Beltangady M, Newton W Jr, Wharam M: Lymphatic metastases with childhood rhabdomyosarcoma. Cancer 60:910–915, 1987.
3. Lawrence W Jr, Hays DM, Moon TE: Lymphatic metastasis with childhood rhabdomyosarcoma. Cancer 39:556–559, 1977.

4. Vezeridis MP, Moore R, Karakousis CP: Metastatic patterns in soft-tissue sarcomas. Arch Surg 118:915–918, 1983.
5. Abbas JS, Holyoke ED, Moore R, Karakousis CP: The surgical treatment and outcome of soft-tissue sarcoma. Arch Surg 116:765–769, 1981.
6. Rizzoni WE, Pass HI, Wesley MN, Rosenberg SA, Roth JA: Resection of recurrent pulmonary metastases in patients with soft-tissue sarcomas. Arch Surg 121:1248–1252, 1986.
7. Udelsman R, Roth JA, Lees D, Jelenich SE, Pass HI: Endobronchial metastases from soft tissue sarcoma. J Surg Oncol 32:145–149, 1986.
8. Bertelsen CA, Eilber FR: Paraneoplastic syndromes with soft-tissue sarcoma: a report of two unusual cases. J Surg Oncol 24:170–172, 1983.
9. Lindell MM Jr, Wallace S, de Santos LA, Bernardino ME: Diagnostic technique for the evaluation of the soft tissue sarcoma. Semin Oncol 8:160–171, 1981.
10. Totty WG: Radiographic evaluation of soft-tissue sarcomas. Orthop Rev 14:257–269, 1985.
11. Bernardino ME, Jing BS, Thomas JL, Lindell MM, Zornozo J: The extremity soft-tissue lesion: a comparative study of ultrasound computed tomography and xeroradiography. Radiology 139:53–59, 1981.
12. Lee KR, Cox GG, Price HI, Johnson JA, Neff JR: Intraarterial digital subtraction arteriographic evaluation of extremity tumors: comparison with conventional arteriography. Radiology 158:255–258, 1986.
13. Enneking W, Chew FS, Springfield DS, Hudson TM, Spanier SS: The role of radionuclide bone-scanning in determining the resectability of soft-tissue sarcomas. J Bone Joint Surg 63-A:249–257, 1981.
14. Hudson TM, Schakel M, Springfield DS, Spanier SS, Enneking WF: The comparative value of bone scintigraphy and computed tomography in determining bone involvement by soft-tissue sarcomas. J Bone Joint Surg 66-A:1400–1407, 1984.
15. Finn HA, Simon MA, Martin WB, Darakjian H: Scintigraphy with gallium-67 citrate in staging of soft-tissue sarcomas of the extremity. J Bone Joint Surg 69-A:886–891, 1987.
16. Hoefnagel CA, Voûte PA, de Kraker J, Behrendt H: Scintigraphic detection of rhabdomyosarcoma. Lancet 1:921, 1987.
17. Lange TA, Austin CW, Seibert JJ, Angtuaco TL, Yandow DR: Ultrasound imaging as a screening study for malignant soft-tissue tumors. J Bone Joint Surg [Am] 69:100–105. 1987.
18. Von Grabbe E, Heller M, Böcker W: Computertomographie bei Weichteilsarkomen. Fortschr Rontgenstr 131:372–378, 1979.
19. Golding SJ, Husband JE: The role of computed tomography in the management of soft tissue sarcomas. Br J Radiol 55:740–747, 1982.
20. Neifeld JP, Walsh JW, Lawrence W Jr: Computed tomography in the management of soft tissue tumors. Surg Gynecol Obstet 155:535–540, 1982.
21. Weekes RG, McLeod RA, Reiman HM, Pritchard DJ: CT of soft-tissue neoplasms. AJR 144:335–360, 1985.
22. Coleman BG, Mulhern CB, Arger PH, Mahboubi S, Chatten J, Kressel HY, Metzger RA: New observations of soft tissue sarcomas with contrast medium-enhanced computed tomography. J Comput Tomogr 9:187–193, 1985.
23. Egund N, Ekelund L, Sako M, Persson B: CT of soft-tissue tumors AJR 137:725–729, 1981.
24. Hudson TM, Schakel M, Springfield DS: Limitations of computed tomography following excisional biopsy of soft tissue sarcomas. Skeletal Radiol 13:49–54, 1985.
25. Totty WG, Murphy WA, Lee JKT: Soft-tissue tumors: MR imaging. Radiology 160:135–141, 1986.
26. Dooms GC, Hricak H, Sollitto RA, Higgins CB: Lipomatous tumors and tumors with fatty component: MR imaging potential and comparison of MR and CT results. Radiology 157:479–483, 1985.
27. Beltran J, Simon DC, Katz W, Weis LD: Increased MR signal intensity in skeletal muscle adjacent to malignant tumors: pathologic correlation and clinical relevance. Radiology 162:251–255, 1987.
28. Hudson TM, Hamlin DJ, Enneking WF, Pettersson H: Magnetic resonance imaging of bone

36

and soft-tissue tumors: early experience in 31 patients compared with computed tomography. Skeletal Radiol 13:134–146, 1985.

29. Aisen AM, Martel W, Braunstein EM, McMillin KI, Phillips WA, Kling TF: MRI and CT evaluation of primary bone and soft-tissue tumors. AJR 146:749–756, 1986.
30. Zimmer WD, Berquist ThH, McLeod RA, Sim FH, Pritchard DJ, Shives ThC, Wold LE, May GR: Bone tumors: magnetic resonance imaging versus computed tomography. Radiology 155:709–718, 1985.
31. Cohen MD, Weetman RM, Provisor AJ, Grosfeld JL, West KW, Cory DA, Smith JA, McGuire W: Efficacy of magnetic resonance imaging in 139 children with tumors. Arch Surg 121:522–529, 1986.
32. Posin JP, Ortendahl DA, Hylton NM, Kaufman L, Watts JC, Crooks LE, Mills CM: Variable magnetic resonance imaging parameters: effect on detection and characterization of lesions. Radiology 155:719–725, 1985.
33. Mizuta H, Yamasaki M: Nuclear magnetic resonance studies on human bone and soft tissue tumors. J Jpn Orthop Assoc 58:97–106, 1984.
34. Mountford CE, May GL, Williams PhG, Tattersall MHN, Russell P, Saunders JK, Holmes KT, Fox RM, Barr JB, Smith ICP: Classifications of human tumours by high resolution magnetic resonance spectroscopy. Lancet 1:651–653, 1986.
35. Oberhaensli RD, Bore PJ, Rampling RP, Hilton-Jones D, Hands LJ, Radda GK: Biochemical investigation of human tumours in vivo with phosphorus-31 magnetic resonance spectroscopy. Lancet 2:8–11, 1986.
36. Weber RS, Benjamin RS, Peters LJ, Ro JY, Achon O, Goepfert H: Soft tissue sarcomas of the head and neck in adolescents and adults. Am J Surg 152:386–392, 1986.
37. Holtz F, Magielski K: Synovial sarcomas of the tongue base. Arch Otolaryngol 111:271–272, 1985.
38. Mamelle G, Richard J, Luboinski B, Schwaab G, Eschwege F, Micheau C: Synovial sarcoma of the head and neck: an account of four cases and review of the literature. Eur J Surg Oncol 12:347–349, 1986.
39. Del Balso AM, Pyatt RS, Busch RF, Hirokawa R, Fink CS: Synovial cell sarcoma of the temporomandibular joint. Arch Otolaryngol 108:520–522, 1982.
40. Hacihanefioglu U, Öztürk AS: Sarcomas of the larynx. Ann Otol Rhinol Laryngol 92:81–84, 1983.
41. Ferlito A, Nicolai P, Caruso G: Angiosarcoma of the larynx. Ann Otol Rhinol Laryngol 94:93–95, 1985.
42. Dodd-O JM, Wieneke KF, Rosman PM: Laryngeal rhabdomyosarcoma. Cancer 59:1012–1018, 1987.
43. Eavey R, Weber AL, Healy G: Rhabdomyosarcoma of the nasopharynx. Ann Otol 91:230–231, 1982.
44. Grant GD, Shields JA, Flanagan JG, Horowitz P: The ultrasonographic and radiologic features of a histologically proven case of alveolar soft-part sarcoma of the orbit. Am J Ophthalmol 87:773–777, 1979.
45. Kuten A, Sapir D, Cohen Y, Haim N, Borovik R, Robinson E: Postirradiation soft tissue sarcoma occurring in breast cancer patients: report of seven cases and results of combination chemotherapy. J Surg Oncol 28:168–171, 1985.
46. Callery CD, Rosen PP, Kinne DW: Sarcoma of the breast. Ann Surg 201:527–532, 1984.
47. Savage R: The treatment of angiosarcoma of the breast. J Surg Oncol 18:129–134, 1981.
48. Khanna S, Gupta S, Khanna NN: Sarcomas of the breast: homogenous or heterogenous? J Surg Oncol 18:119–128, 1981.
49. Solla JA, Reed K: Primary retroperitoneal sarcomas. Am J Surg 152:496–498, 1986.
50. Kristofferson AO, Domellöf L, Emdin SO, Kullenberg K: Malignant fibrous histiocytoma of the gallbladder: a case report. J Surg Oncol 23:56–59, 1983.
51. Sarma DP, Weilbaecher TG: Retroperitoneal malignant fibrous histiocytoma presenting with inferior vena caval obstruction. J Surg Oncol 32:153–155, 1986.
52. Chen KTK: Malignant fibrous histiocytoma of the kidney. J Surg Oncol 27:248–250, 1984.

53. Simansky DA, Schiby G, Dreznik Z, Jacob ET: Rapid progressive dissemination of hemangiosarcoma of the spleen following spontaneous rupture. World J Surg 10:142–145, 1986.
54. McGrath PC, Neifeld JP, Lawrence W Jr, DeMay RM, Kay S, Shelton Horsley J, Parker GA: Improved survival following complete excision of retroperitoneal sarcomas. Ann Surg 200:200–204, 1984.
55. Bedikian AY, Khankhanian N, Valdivieso M, Heilbrun LK, Benjamin RS, Yap BS, Nelson RS, Bodey GP: Sarcoma of the stomach: clinicopathologic study of 43 cases. J Surg Oncol 13:121–127, 1980.
56. Schneider K, Dickerhoff R, Bertele RM: Malignant gastric sarcoma: diagnosis by ultrasound and endoscopy. Pediatr Radiol 16:69–70, 1986.
57. Golding RP, van Zanten TEG, Kwee WS: CT in palpable non-obstructing intestinal tumors. J Belge Radiol 66:447–452, 1983.
58. Chiotasso PJP, Fazio VW: Prognostic factors of 28 leiomyosarcomas of the small intestine. Surg Gynecol Obstet 155:197–202, 1982.
59. Walker MJ, Wood DK, Briele HA, Greager JA, Patel M, Das Gupta TK: Soft tissue sarcomas of the distal extremities. Surgery 99:392–398, 1986.
60. Orson GG, Sim FH, Reiman HM, Taylor WF: Liposarcoma of the musculoskeletal system. Cancer 60:1362–1370, 1987.
61. Lehti PM, Stephens Moseley H, Peetz ME, Fletcher WS: Liposarcoma of the leg. Am J Surg 144:44–47, 1982.
62. Lieberman PH, Foote FW, Stewart FW, Berg JW: Alveolar soft-part sarcoma. JAMA 198:1047–1051, 1966.
63. Randall Radin D, Ralls PW, Boswell WD, Lundell C, Halls JM: Alveolar soft part sarcoma: CT findings. J Comput Assist Tomogr 8:344–345, 1984.
64. Chung EB, Enzinger FM: Extraskeletal osteosarcoma. Cancer 60:1132–1142, 1987.
65. Weinberger G, Levinsohn EM: Computed tomography in the evaluation of sarcomatous tumors of the thigh. AJR 130:115–118, 1978.
66. Laursen K, Reiter S: Computed tomography in soft tissue disorders of the lower extremities. Acta Orthop Scand 51:881–885, 1980.
67. Levine E: Computed tomography of musculoskeletal tumors. CRC Critical Reviews in Diagnostic Imagery 16:279–309, 1981.
68. Enneking WF, Spanier SS, Goodman MA: A system for the surgical staging of musculoskeletal sarcoma. Clin Orthop 153:106–120, 1980.
69. Waag KL, Gerein V, Kornhuber B, Katsch P, Treuner J: Synovial sarcoma in childhood. Kinderchirz 39:48–50, 1984.
70. Israels SJ, Chan HSL, Daneman A, Weitzman SS: Synovial sarcoma in childhood. AJR 142:803–806, 1984.
71. Petasnick JP, Turner DA, Charters JR, Gitelis S, Zacharias CE: Soft-tissue masses of the locomotor system: comparison of MR imaging with CT. Radiology 160:125–133, 1986.
72. Nidecker AC, Müller S, Aue WP, Seelig J, Fridrich F, Remagen W, Hartweg H, Benz UF: Extremity bone tumors: evaluation by P-31 MR spectroscopy. Radiology 157:167–174, 1985.
73. Treu EBWM, de Slegte RGM, Golding RP, Sperber M, van Zanten TEG, Valk J: CT findings in paravertebral synovial sarcoma. J Comput Assit Tomogr 10:460–462, 1986.
74. Van Zanten TEG, Golding RP: CT and MR demonstration of leiomyosarcoma of inferior vena cava. J Comput Assist Tomogr 11:670–674, 1987.

3. Musculoskeletal tumor staging: 1988 update

Wiliam F. Enneking

The Musculoskeletal Tumor Society (MTS) staging system

Since 1960, prospective primary observational data have been gathered and stored on primary benign and malignant neoplasms of the musculoskeletal system in the W. Thaxton Springfield Study Center at the University of Florida. In 1974, based upon analysis of this data, a staging system for primary malignant tumors of connective tissue histogenesis was constructed together with definitions of oncologic surgical margins and oncologic surgical procedures. By 1979, 258 cases had been staged and enough time had passed to evaluate the system. At that time, the Musculoskeletal Tumor Society (MTS) contributed an additional 139 cases from 13 member institutions to form an initial study group of 397 cases.

After analysis of the data, the system was modified to the form first published in 1980 [1]. Because of the emphasis placed on correlating the system with surgical margins and procedures, it was termed a surgical staging system and was based on three factors: grade (G), anatomic site (T), and metastases (M).

Grade was subdivided into low grade (G_1) or high grade (G_2) on a combination of histologic and radiographic criteria. Before selecting this two-grade system, both three- and four-grade systems were considered.

The four-grade system described by Broders et al. [2] for soft tissue fibrosarcomas was based on histologic criteria originally applied to carcinomas and many of the criteria were not widely applicable to sarcomas of both bone and soft tissue.

A three-grade system described by Evans et al. [3] and Sanerkin [4] for chondrosarcomas and by Enzinger et al. [5] for soft tissue sarcomas was also examined. The criteria for bone and soft tissue lesions were quite disparate, did not take into account radiographic criteria, and did not facilitate the principal objective of the system—surgical planning. In the nomenclature of surgical margins (intracapsular, marginal, wide, and radical) used to stratify surgical procedures—both limb-salvage resections and amputations—the data indicated that there were only two margins that obtained adequate local control—wide and radical. Both intracapsular and marginal margins resulted

Pinedo, H.M., Verweij, J., eds. TREATMENT OF SOFT TISSUE SARCOMAS.

in unacceptably high recurrence rates. As there was no intermediate surgical margin to correlate with an intermediate-grade lesion, a three-grade system was discarded in favor of a two-grade system with both histologic and radiographic criteria.

Anatomic site was subdivided into intracompartmental (A) or extracompartmental (B) location based upon radiographic and surgical criteria that demonstrated whether the lesion was confined within well-defined anatomic compartments (bone, joint, intramuscular compartments), bounded by the natural barriers to tumor extension (cortical bone, articular cartilage, joint capsule, major fascial septae). Although size was recognized as a significant variable of the anatomic site, it was not included as a criteria because it did not form a basis for surgical planning. The determinant surgical criteria of the anatomic site was the involvement of the major neurovascular structures. This was best accounted for by compartmentalization and virtually ignored by size.

On the other hand, the prognostic significance of size was accounted for in the system by the close correlation between size and compartmentalization— i.e., the great preponderance of small lesions were intracompartmental and the large lesions were virtually all extracompartmental.

The third factor, metastasis, was expressed as clinically present (M_1) or absent (M_0). The data demonstrated that there was no difference in the prognosis in those cases in which there was regional lymph node metastasis (N) and those in which distant metastases were present (M). Thus, both were combined into a single criteria.

The fine details of this surgical staging system were published in 1980 and are summarized below:

G_1 Low grade malignant
G_2 High grade malignant

T_1 Intracompartmental
T_2 Extracompartmental

M_0 No metastasis
M_1 Metastasis

Stage I
   A $G_1 T_1 M_0$
   B $G_1 T_2 M_0$
Stage II
   A $G_2 T_1 M_0$
   B $G_2 T_2 M_0$
Stage III
   A $G_{1-2} T_{1-2} M_1$

Analysis of the data in 1980 showed that there was a stepwise difference in prognosis for each progression in the system. These differences were the same whether the lesions were staged intramurally or extramurally, or whether the lesions had originated in bone or soft tissue. At this point in time, the MTS adopted the system for its institutional protocols and studies. It has been widely adopted in the literature for staging both bone and soft tissue lesions and has been used as the staging system for the 1983, 1985, and 1987 international symposia on limb salvage [6, 7].

In 1986, after greater experience with the system, the criteria for compartmentalization were clarified and an extension of the system to allow staging of benign lesions was presented [8]. In this extension, grade was further subdivided into G_0 (benign), G_1 (low-grade malignant), and G_2 (high-grade malignant). The criteria for anatomic site was similarly extended into T_0 (intracapsular), T_1 (extracapsular, intracompartmental), and T_2 (extracapsular, extracompartmental). In addition, the term intracapsular was substituted for intralesional as a surgical margin. This 1986 format represents the current surgical staging system of the MTS and is summarized below:

G_0 Benign
G_1 Low grade malignant
G_2 High grade malignant
T_0 Intracapsular
T_1 Extracapsular, intracompartmental
T_2 Extracapsular, extracompartmental
M_0 No metastasis
M_1 Metastasis

Benign
Stage 1 $G_0 \, T_0 \, M_0$
Stage 2 $G_0 \, T_1 \, M_0$
Stage 3 $G_0 \, T_2 \, M_{0-1}$

Malignant
Stage I
  A $G_1 \, T_1 \, M_0$
  B $G_1 \, T_2 \, M_0$
Stage II
  A $G_2 \, T_1 \, M_0$
  B $G_2 \, T_2 \, M_0$
Stage III
  A $G_{1-2} \, T_{1-2} \, M_1$

The American Joint Commission (AJC) staging system

At about the same time that the MTS surgical system was developing, the American Joint Commission for Cancer Staging and End Results Reporting

(AJC) had formed two independent task forces charged with the responsibility for developing separate staging systems for bone and soft tissue sarcomas.

The Task Force on Bone reported in 1977 that they had failed to devise a satisfactory system and recommended that "institutions with access to large numbers of patients, consistency in management, and long-term follow-up undertake this task" [9]. This is what was done at the University of Florida and evolved into the MTS system. The next report of the AJC Bone Task Force in 1985 was the recommendation that the AJC adopt the criteria for G, T, and M of the MTS system, but, in order to conform to the four-stage format, the AJC modified the numbering of the stages [10]. In this modification, Stages I and II remained synonymous with those of the MTS, Stage III was left undefined, and Stage IV of the ACJ bone system was the same as Stage III of the MTS system. The 1985 AJC surgical staging system for bone is listed below:

G_1 Low grade malignant
G_2 High grade malignant

T_1 Intracompartmental
T_2 Extracompartmental

M_0 No metastasis
M_1 Metastasis

Stage I
  A $G_1 \, T_1 \, M_0$
  B $G_1 \, T_2 \, M_0$
Stage II
  A $G_2 \, T_1 \, M_0$
  B $G_2 \, T_2 \, M_0$
Stage III
  A $G_{1-2} \, T_{1-2} \, M_1$

Thus, although the criteria and stratification were the same in both systems, the nomenclature was different. The other minor difference was that the MTS system, being confined to lesions of connective tissue histogenesis, excluded Ewing's sarcoma while the AJC bone system specifically included it. Since 1985, the AJC bone system has not been widely used in the literature.

The AJC Soft Tissue Task Force in 1977 published a proposed system for staging soft tissue lesions [11]. This system was markedly different from either the AJC bone or the combined MTS system. It was a four-stage system based upon histologic grade (G); size and/or invasion of bone, artery, or nerve (T); nodal metastases (N); and distant metastases (M).

Grade was subdivided into three grades; low grade (G), moderate grade (G_2), and high grade (G_3). In addition, certain histogenic types (synovial sarcoma, angiosarcoma, and rhabdomyosarcoma) were arbitrarily assigned to the high-grade group irrespective of the histologic criteria as if those lesions never were of low or intermediate grade.

T was subdivided by two criteria, by size in the lower stages and by whether or not the lesion invaded bone, artery, or nerve in the higher grades. T_1 was assigned to lesions <5 cm and T_2 to lesions >5 cm in size. T_3 was assigned to lesions that invaded bone, artery, or nerve.

Metastasis was subdivided by regional node involvement (N) or distant metastasis (M). N_0 signified no node involvement, and N_1 signified metastatic node involvement. Similarly M_0 and M_1 signified the absence or presence of distant metastasis. These criteria were used to construct the 1977 four-stage AJC system for soft tissue sarcoma, listed below:

G_1 Low grade malignant
G_2 Moderate grade malignant
G_3 High grade malignant

T_1 <5 cm
T_2 >5 cm
T_3 Involves bone, artery, nerve

N_0 No node metastasis
N_1 Node metastasis

M_0 No distant metastasis
M_1 Distant metastasis

Stage I
a $G_1 \, T_1 \, N_0 \, M_0$
b $G_1 \, T_2 \, N_0 \, M_0$
Stage II
a $G_2 \, T_1 \, N_0 \, M_0$
b $G_2 \, T_2 \, N_0 \, M_0$
Stage III
a $G_3 \, T_1 \, N_0 \, M_0$
b $G_3 \, T_2 \, N_0 \, M_0$
c $G_{1-3} \, T_{1-2} \, N_1 \, M_0$
Stage IV
a $G_{1-3} \, T_3 \, N_{0-1} \, M_0$
b $G_{1-3} \, T_{1-3} \, N_{0-1} \, M_1$

The first three stages were stratified by histologic grade and subdivided on the basis of size alone. In Stage III, a third subdivision was added for lesions with nodal metastasis. Stage IV was subdivided into two groups, the first with invasion of bone, artery, or nerve, and the second on the basis of distant metastasis. Analysis of the data from 423 verified cases showed a stepwise progression in prognosis for each stage, but no difference between the subdivisions in the stages based on size; those lesions placed in Stage III on the basis of node metastasis had a worse prognosis than those placed in Stage IV on the basis of bone, artery, or nerve invasion.

The system has not been widely used in the ensuing decade. The principal reasons for its lack of utilization appeared to be its complexity leading to poor compliance, its inconsistencies, and the difficulties in correlating the stages with surgical planning.

Some examples of inconsistencies include: assigning a higher stage to a small, superficial, low-grade synovial sarcoma (Stage IIIa) than to a large, deep, moderate-grade liposarcoma (Stage IIb); or assigning a higher stage to a small, low-grade fibrosarcoma invading bone (Stabe IVa) than to a larger, high-grade malignant fibrous histiocytoma with lymph node metastasis (Stage IIIc)

Recognizing these shortcomings, the AJC Soft Tissue Task Force has recently recommended several modifications to the system (H.L. Suit, personal communication). The recommendation, as yet unpublished, removes bone, artery, and nerve invasion as a criteria for T, removes histogenic type as a criteria for G, and places both node and distant metastasis in the same stage. Stages I, II, and III are determined by grade and subdivided by size while Stage IV represents metastasis subdivided by node and distant metastasis. The 1987 AJC modified staging system for soft tissue sarcoma is listed below:

G_1 Low grade malignant
G_2 Moderate grade malignant
G_3 High grade malignant

T_1 <5 cm
T_2 >5 cm

N_0 No node metastasis
N_1 Node metastasis

M_0 No distant metastasis
M_1 Distant metastasis

Stage I
A $G_1 \, T_1 \, N_0 \, M_0$
B $G_1 \, T_2 \, N_0 \, M_0$
Stage II
A $G_2 \, T_1 \, N_0 \, M_0$
B $G_2 \, T_2 \, N_0 \, M_0$
Stage III
A $G_3 \, T_1 \, N_0 \, M_0$
B $G_3 \, T_2 \, N_0 \, M_0$
Stage IV
A $G_{1-3} \, T_{1-2} \, N_1 \, M_0$
B $G_{1-3} \, T_{1-2} \, N_{0-1} \, M_1$

These modifications make this system less complex and remove the majority of the inconsistencies from the original version.

Discussion

At present, there are three different staging systems for bone and soft tissue sarcomas:

1. The MTS system for both bone and soft tissue sarcomas
2. The AJC bone system
3. The modified AJC soft tissue system

The MTS System has the advantages of simplicity, a high degree of compliance, wide understanding and international usage, ease of correlation with surgical planning, and the same criteria for both bone and soft tissue lesions.

The AJC bone system is virtually the same as the MTS system. It has not been widely publicized and is virtually unknown outside of the AJC Task Force. The inconsistency of assigning metastatic disease to Stage IV in one system and to Stage III in another system leads to confusion. On the other hand, there is value in uniformity in formulating the various staging systems for different classes of malignancy wherein Stage IV always represents distant metastasis.

The AJC soft tissue system, as originally proposed, differed markedly from the other two systems. The modifications simplifying the system and removing the inconsistencies brings it into closer alignment with the other two systems.

In view of the recent modifications of both the AJC bone and AJC soft tissue systems, this would seem to be a propitious moment to consider combining the three into a unified whole by examining the differences in criteria for each of the factors and attempting to reconcile the differences.

G (histologic grade)

Both systems for bone use a two-grade system for malignant lesions while the AJC soft tissue system uses a three-grade system. The two-grade system places the clearly low- and high-grade lesions in two separate stages and requires the selection of one or the other stages for lesions with intermediate histologic characteristics. This selection is enhanced by data from clinical, radiographic, and specialized imaging techniques that are considered along with the histologic criteria [8]. In the era in which it was devised, when surgery alone was the usual method of treatment, the two-grade format correlated well with surgical planning. Low-grade lesions were well managed with procedures obtaining wide margins and the selection between resection and amputation correlated well with whether the lesion was situated intra- or extracompartmentally. High-grade lesions required procedures that obtained radical margins and, again, the selection of resection versus amputation to obtain a radical margin correlated well the anatomic setting of the lesion.

The three-grade system also allows the clearly low- and high-grade lesions to be placed in separate stages, but adds another stage for intermediate-grade lesions. While the criteria for the gradation are purely histologic and do not take into account radiographic or specialized imaging data, criteria for the three-grade system have been published both for some bone lesions, notably chondrosarcoma [3, 4], and for soft tissue sarcomas [5]. These criteria are widely understood and applied by pathologists. Of considerable significance is the potential for flow cytometry and similar techniques to increase the accuracy of histologic grading.

Correlation between a three-grade system and surgical planning offers a wider range of surgical options than does the two-grade system. In this era of combining marginal, wide, and occasionally radical margins with pre- and postoperative adjuvant modalities, a three-grade system appears to offer potentially better therapeutic correlations than does a two-stage system.

Both systems have shown significant differences in prognosis between the stages based on either the two- or three-grade system.

In sum, there does not appear to be a clear-cut advantage of one system over the other. Those whose perspective is primarily surgical appear to prefer the two-grade system and those whose perspective is primarily pathologic favor the three-grade system.

T (site and/or size)

Site and/or size are determined by different criteria in the MTS and AJC soft tissue systems while they are the same between the MTS and AJC bone systems. In the MTS and AJC bone systems, T is used to designate the anatomic site and is subdivided into intracompartmentally (T_1) and extracompartmentally (T_2) situated lesions. In the modified AJC soft tissue system, T is stratified by size <5 cm (T_1) or >5 cm (T_2). There are cogent reasons for favoring compartmentalization over size as the criterion for subdividing T. The anatomic setting of a lesion is the key determinant in surgical planning while size per se is not. Compartmentalization has both anatomic and functional implications while size does not. With current imaging techniques, compartmentalization can be precisely determined and is recorded for reproducibility. Size changes from a wet to dry specimen, from the radiographic image to the operating room, and from the operating room to the pathology suite. Compartmentalization takes into account size, while size alone does not taken into account compartmentalization. While, in the original AJC soft tissue system, compartmentalization was indirectly accounted for, albeit somewhat awkwardly; in the modified system, it is ignored in favor of size alone. While it is true that size is related to prognosis, it is almost a linear progression until 20 cm. Thus, although lesions >5 cm have a worse prognosis than lesions

<5 cm, the same can be said for 8, 10, 12, or 15 cm as the dividing line. This, in all likelihood, accounts for why there is little prognostic significance to a two-step division in T on the basis of any one size.

In sum, there is a clear-cut advantage to using the concept of compartmentalization over that of size as the criterion for T.

M (metastasis)

Metastasis is treated the same by the AJC bone and the MTS systems by combining nodal and distant metastases into a single M. However, the AJC bone system calls this Stage IV and leaves Stage III unnamed because, in other AJC systems, stage II is reserved for metastatic disease. In the modified AJC soft tissue system, metastases are subdivided into nodal (N) and distant (M) and placed as subdivisions of Stage IV. In their 1977 report, the AJC Soft Tissue Task Force had nodal metastasis as Stage IIIc and distant metastasis as Stage IVb. There was no difference in prognosis between these two stages. Be that as it may, there does not seem to be a compelling reason to favor separating or combining nodal and distant metastases. Combining them, as in the AJC bone and MTS systems is simpler, while separating them as in the AJC soft tissue system may, with more cases, provide a significant stratification to Stage IV.

Conclusions

It is evident that having a single system for both bone and soft tissue lesions would be better than the current multiple systems. The alternatives are to adopt universally the three-stage combined MTS system, reconcile the differences into a combined four-stage system, or continue with the current situation. The later alternative is the least desirable. Any reconciliation should logically be based upon the most useful criteria for G, T, and M.

As to grade, the three-step system appears preferable. Grading into low, moderate, and high is widely practiced by pathologists, and a three-step system will in all likelihood better accommodate future diagnostic and therapeutic developments.

Clearly, the anatomic localization of the lesion is the preferable criterion for subdividing T. The rapid advances in radiography and specialized imaging techniques continue to increase the resolution by which compartmentalization can be determined.

The presence of metastasis should be expressed in a single stage and it would seem preferable to designate both regional and distant metastases as subsets.

For the advantages of uniformity, a four-stage, three-grade format in which T is determined by compartmentalization and M is subdivided into N and M combines the better features of the three systems. The 1987 unified system is shown below:

G_1 Low grade malignant
G_2 Moderate grade malignant
G_3 High grade malignant

T_1 Intracompartmental
T_2 Extracompartmental

N_0 No node metastasis
N_1 Node metastasis

M_0 No distant metastasis
M_1 Distant metastasis

Stage I
A $G_1 T_1 N_0 M_0$
B $G_1 T_2 N_0 M_0$
Stage II
A $G_2 T_1 N_0 M_0$
B $G_2 T_2 N_0 M_0$
Stage III
A $G_3 T_1 N_0 M_0$
B $G_3 T_2 N_0 M_0$
Stage IV
A $G_{1-3} T_{1-2} N_1 M_0$
B $G_{1-3} T_{1-2} N_{0-1} M_1$

There is no doubt that conversion from either the current widely used three-stage MTS system or the AJC systems to a four-stage unified system would cause serious burdens to those individuals, institutions, and interinstitutional groups whose protocols and data storage are based on one of the current systems. Whether conversion to a unified (modified combined) four-stage system is worth the price of these burdens is the heart of the matter. However, there is no question that universal adoption of one or the other of these systems would be a significant step forward in musculoskeletal oncology.

References

1. Enneking WF, Spanier SS, Goodman MA: A system for the surgical staging of musculo-skeletal sarcoma. Clin Orthop 153:106–120, 1980.
2. Broders AC, Hargrave R, Myerding HW: Pathologic features of soft tissue fibrosarcoma. Surg Gynecol Obstet 69:267–280, 1939.
3. Evans HL, Ayala AG, Romsdahl MM: Prognostic factors in chondrosarcoma of bone: a clinico-pathologic analysis with emphasis on histologic grading. Cancer 40:818, 1977.
4. Sanerkin NG: The diagnosis and grading of chondrosarcoma of bone. Cancer 45:582–594, 1980.

5. Enzinger FM, Lattes R, Tartoni H: Histologic typing of soft tissue tumors. Geneva: World Health Organization, 1969.
6. Enneking WF (ed): Limb salvage in musculoskeletal oncology. New York: Churchill Livingstone, 1987.
7. Kotz R. (ed): Proceedings of the 2nd international meeting on the design and application of tumor prosthesis for bone and joint reconstruction. Vienna: Egermann, 1983.
8. Enneking WF: A system of staging musculoskeletal neoplasms. Clin Orthop 204:9–24, 1986.
9. Copeland MM, Robbins GF, Myers MN: Development of a clinical staging system for primary malignant tumors of bone: a progress report. In: Management of primary bone and soft tissue tumors. Chicago: Year Book Medical, 1977, p 35.
10. Hutter R, Bears O, Henson D, Myers M: Manual for staging of cancer, 3rd edn. Philadelphia: JB Lippincott, 1985.
11. Russell WW, Cohen J, Enzinger F, Hajdn SI, Heise H, Martin RG, Meissner W, Miller WT, Schmitz RL, Suit HD: A clinical and pathologic staging system for soft tissue sarcomas. Cancer 40:1562, 1977.

4. Surgery of soft tissue sarcomas

G. Westbury

The aim of local treatment of soft tissue sarcomas is complete eradication of the primary tumor. Regional lymph node metastasis is uncommon, being detected in only 2.7% in the series reported by Lindberg et al. [1] and in 4% of the author's cases at initial presentation. Surgical resection with microscopically free margins is the most certain single method of local control [2–4]. The addition of radiotherapy to surgery improves the rate of local control [1, 5]. It has been suggested that cytotoxic therapy contributes to local control, whether given systemically [6] or by the regional intra-arterial route [7, 8], but further evaluation of these claims is required. Since surgery, radiotherapy, and chemotherapy are often used in complementary fashion, joint consultation among surgeon, radiation oncologist, and medical oncologist is essential.

The principles underlying the surgery of soft tissue sarcomas are the same whatever the histological type or grade; therefore, the different pathological categories are not separately discussed in this chapter. The operative approach is determined rather by the surgical pathology of this tumor group within the context of the anatomical region involved [9].

Pathological anatomy in relation to local treatment

Inspection of a soft tissue sarcoma with the naked eye usually gives the impression of encapsulation, which tempts the unwary surgeon to simple enucleation. This apparent capsule is, however, infiltrated by tumor cells and such a "shell-out" procedure, without further treatment, is followed by an extremely high risk of local failure. Soft tissue sarcomas are slow to invade fascia, periosteum, epineurium, or the adventitia of major arteries. Spread away from the site of origin is along the lines of least tissue resistance, parallel to fascial planes and between muscle bundles, sometimes producing skip lesions at a distance from the main tumor mass. In the limbs, this spread is in the long axis.

Enneking et al. [9] have classified operations for soft tissue sarcoma on this basis for any anatomical site. A *radical operation* removes the entire musculofascial compartment in which the tumor and its potential skip lesions lie. *Wide*

Pinedo, H.M., Verweij, J., eds. TREATMENT OF SOFT TISSUE SARCOMAS.
© Kluwer Academic Publishers, Boston. ISBN: 0-89838-391-9. All rights reserved.

resection implies clearance with a generous margin, but does not encompass the entire compartment. *Marginal resection* means enucleation in the plane of the pseudocapsule; even when the tumor is exposed over a small segment of its surface, the procedure should be classified as marginal. In *intracapsular (intralesional) excision*, the tumor is debulked and macroscopic disease remains. The validity of these concepts is supported by the reported data for local failure according to the extent of surgery used as the sole method of treatment, e.g., marginal, 90%; wide, 39%; and radical, 25% [1]. These figures are significantly reduced by adjuvant radiotherapy.

The surgical ideal of compartmental resection cannot always be achieved. Many sarcomas arise outside a well-defined compartment and tumors that were originally intracompartmental can extend to penetrate beyond these confines. In the limbs, the popliteal and antecubital fossae, the femoral triangle, and the axilla lack a complete fascial investment and, short of radical amputation, surgery can at best only be wide. Adjuvant irradiation is therefore often required to minimize the risk of local failure. Similarly the subcutaneous and retroperitoneal spaces are loosely textured, open regions. Subcutaneously situated tumors can usually be widely excised or radiotherapy given when the margins of clearance are unsatisfactory. By contrast, wide resection is often impossible in the retroperitoneum, and the dose of irradiation is limited by tolerance of the viscera so that local failure is common.

Biopsy

For small, superficial sarcomas, excision biopsy provides the entire specimen for analysis and does not impair subsequent definitive surgery. In the commoner case of the larger, deeply situated tumor, marginal excision can cause considerable difficulty when reexcision is undertaken because the margins of the tumor bed are not known, and postsurgical hematoma, edema, or scarring further obscure the operative field so that total surgical clearance of potentially contaminated tissues may not be possible. Incision biopsy provides ample pathological material and, if well sited, the wound track can readily be included within the final surgical specimen. Even so, Mankin et al. [10] reported complications such as hematoma, infection, and tumor cell spillage in 17.3% of a series of open biopsies for bone and soft tissue tumors. They believed that poor biopsy technique adversely affected outcome in some of their patients in respect to loss of limb and possibly survival. Others have found that neither the performance of a biopsy nor its timing in relation to definitive resection significantly affected local recurrence [2]. Punch biopsy using a trocar and cannula [11] yields ample material with little tissue disturbance, but requires general anesthesia. Kissin et al. have evaluated and compared Tru-cut biopsy [12] and fine-needle aspiration cytology [13]. Tru-cut biopsy produced cores adequate for the diagnosis of sarcoma in 84% of patients, and the predictive accuracy in those specimens was 87%–98%, varying among three independently reporting pathologists. Fine-needle aspiration cytology yielded a higher proportion of inadequate specimens, but the predictive value of a positive diagnosis was still >90%. These cheap and minimally invasive techniques are therefore of value in the outpatient assessment of suspicious masses. They may not, however, allow sufficient precision in tumor grading when pre-surgical adjuvant therapy is under consideration.

Sarcomas of the limbs and limb girdles

Prior to the now widespread acceptance of the value of radiotherapy in combined management [14], amputation was a relatively frequent choice of resection for soft tissue sarcomas of the extremities. As already indicated, not all of these tumors are anatomically suited to radical limb-sparing resection—as classically defined—and the frequency of local failure increases with decreasing tumor margins in the absence of adjuvant therapy. The first major series of patients treated by the combined-modality approach was that of Cade [15], who demonstrated the reduction of local recurrence by irradiation following less than adequate excision. He also reported that limb conservation was associated with a better survival than was amputation, though this might have resulted from case selection. Potter et al. [16] found, as have many others, that amputation achieved a lower local recurrence rate than did limb-sparing management, but in their study there was no difference in disease-free or over-all survival between the two groups. While the incidence of metastasis and death has been associated with local failure by some investigators [17, 18], multivariate analysis of the author's material (A.T. Stotter et al., unpublished) has shown that the incidence of local recurrence has no significant influence on overall outcome, which was predominantly determined by tumor size and grade. The general conclusion is that limb conservation is a justifiable approach and any detriment to survival is a small one. Even after local failure, limb salvage may still be attained by further resection [16], and amputation can be reserved for locally unresectable disease.

Interaction of surgery with radiotherapy

With surgery as the sole treatment modality, local failure is directly related to margins of resection and the surgeon must aim toward radical resection, whether by limb-sparing surgery or amputation. This policy of maximal surgery may be unavoidable when disease recurs following radiotherapy. For the nonirradiated patient, however, the need for classic radical surgery—i.e., compartmental resection where anatomically feasible, removing entire muscle groups and associated major neurovascular structures—has been challenged. Suit et al. [19] advocate no more than wide or marginal resection as determined by the local anatomy, especially proximity of major nerves and vessels. The field at risk in terms of satellite and skip lesions is covered by appropriate irradiation portals. There were only 16 (10.8%) of 148 local failures in this series. Lindberg [20] reported a similar policy of limited surgical excision with maintenance of a functional limb in 84.7% of patients. The value of radiotherapy in support of limited resection is important in the distal parts of the extremities, especially the upper [21], where anatomical constraints seldom permit more than limited resection without serious compromise of function. In the proximal segments of the extremities, sacrifice of entire muscle groups produces surprisingly little functional deficit. An exception is the quadriceps femoris, whose total loss results in instability of the knee; preservation of one head, if not involved by tumor, maintains the ability to lock the joint. Whether surgery should be deliberately restricted in the proximal segments can only be tested by studies in which both local disease control and function are compared.

Conservation surgery for soft tissue sarcomas of the limb girdles can pre-

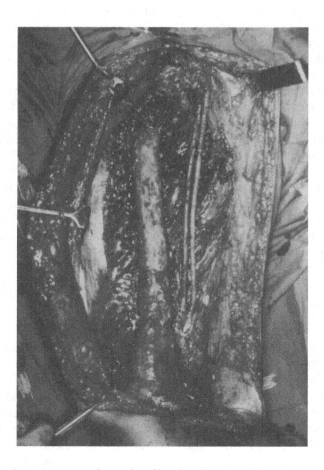

Figure 1. Anterior compartmental resection. Vessels and cortex of femur exposed.

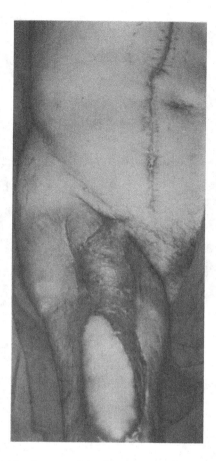

Figure 2. Inferiorly based island rectus abdominis myocutaneous flap for wound breakdown following radiotherapy and compartmental resection. Mesh graft to muscle pedicle.

sent a major technical challenge. Wide soft part resections may be combined with en bloc removal of adjacent involved bone. At the shoulder girdle, useful function of elbow, wrist, and hand is retained even after sacrifice of scapula, clavicle, and head of humerus (Tikhoff–Linberg operation), provided the neurovascular bundle is not involved. For sarcomas of the groin, the surgeon must be prepared to sarcifice and replace skin and major vascular structures, and to provide sound cover (see below).

When sarcoma persists or recurs in an irradiated field, the surgeon has less latitude in conserving major neurovascular structures that lie closely adjacent to the tumor mass. En bloc arterial resection and reconstruction may be required. In deciding whether to sacrifice major nerves or to amputate, the surgeon must judge whether the resulting limb will be more or less useful to the patient than the required prosthesis. In the lower limb, total loss of sciatic

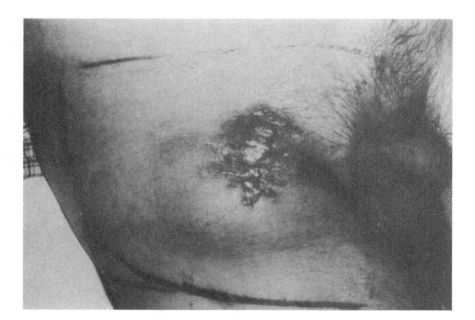

A

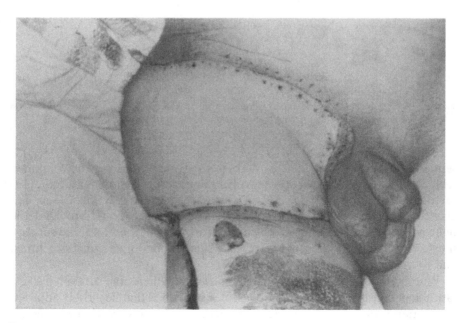

B

Figure 3. (*A*) Fungating sarcoma of groin advancing during radiotherapy. (*B*) Excision and repair with tensor fasciae latae myocutaneous flap. Radiotherapy completed through the flap.

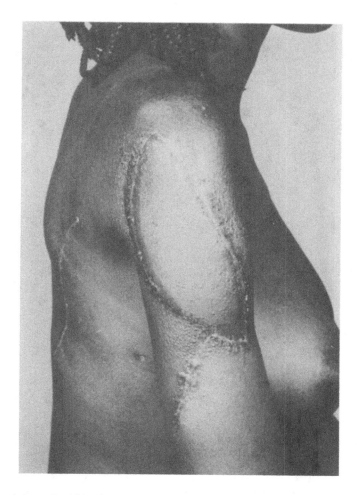

Figure 4. Latissimus dorsi island myocutaneous flap to arm. Primary closure of donor site.

or femoral nerve is compatible with worthwhile function. In the upper limb, loss of the radial nerve is readily offset by splinting or tendon transfer. Sacrifice of median or of ulnar nerve is more disabling, but it must be borne in mind that no prosthesis can match the value of retention, even of limited sensory capacity, in the fingers.

Surgical wound morbidity is increased by radiotherapy whether delivered preoperatively [22] or intraoperatively [23]. Special care must therefore be applied to the blood supply of skin edges and the obliteration of dead space so that per primam healing is achieved. When major arteries have been exposed in the dissection (Fig. 1), or resected and replaced, wound breakdown may lead to secondary hemorrhage and require emergency amputation. These complications should be anticipated and avoided by the use of well-vascularized

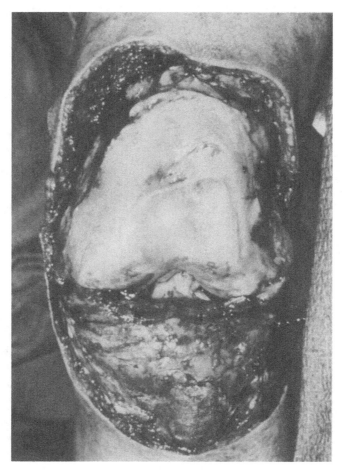

A

Figure 5. (*A*) Exposed knee joint following resection of sarcoma arising in the prepatellar bursa. (*B*) Reconstruction by free microvascular latissimus dorsi myocutaneous flap.

flaps introduced from nonirradiated areas. In the Royal Marsden Hospital series of 180 surgical interventions for sarcomas of the limbs and trunk, flap reconstruction was used in 18 patients (A.T. Stotter et al., unpublished). These included five cutaneous flaps, three muscle transpositions with split skin cover, six myocutaneous flaps (Figs. 2–4), and four free microvascular transfers (Fig. 5A and B). The mobilized greater omentum was used for three further patients in one of whom the limb was successfully salvaged after secondary hemorrhage from the femoral artery. While considerations of wound healing argue in favor of surgery as the initial treatment in the combined approach, preoperative irradiation is of particular value in management of the larger, semifixed tumor that may be rendered more easily resectable.

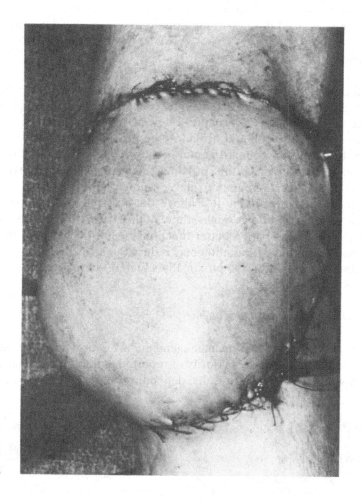

B

Since wound morbidity tends to be greater with larger tumor size and in the elderly [22], this group requires special attention to wound repair.

Interaction with regional chemotherapy

Sarcomas have been treated with cytotoxic drugs via the intra-arterial route using the technique of isolated extracorporeal perfusion [7, 24]. Complete, lasting remission by perfusion alone is exceptional and the addition of surgical resection with or without irradiation is essential to prevent a high local failure rate. It is not clear that this major procedure adds significantly to the benefit achievable by the combination of surgery and radiotherapy. A simpler protocol of intra-arterial doxorubicin, followed by rapid fraction radiotherapy immediately prior to resection, has been more systematically pursued [8]. Local failure occurred in only 4%, but complications of therapy were reported in

35%, half of whom required a second operative procedure. A more recent study using a reduced dose of irradiation awaits further evaluation.

Amputation

Amputation is usually avoidable by multimodality limb-sparing management and, though occasionally indicated as the primary surgical option, it is more often used as a secondary procedure following failure of limb conservation. The site of amputation should ordinarily be proximal to the involved compartment because transcompartmental section runs the risk of stump recurrence (Fig. 6). For sarcomas of the proximal thigh not extending into the pelvis, complete hindquarter amputation may be unnecessary. In such cases, the bone is sectioned horizontally just above the acetabulum; the procedure is technically simpler and the residual stump of iliac bone provides counterpressure for the prosthesis with a better functional result than follows the classic operation. Preoperative irradiation may reduce the incidence of stump failure when primary amputation for proximally situated tumors presents technical difficulties in clearance [22].

Functional and psychological sequelae

These aspects of limb-sparing management have received relatively little attention [19, 25] though the majority of reported patients have been assessed as having good or reasonable results, depending on the criteria of evaluation.

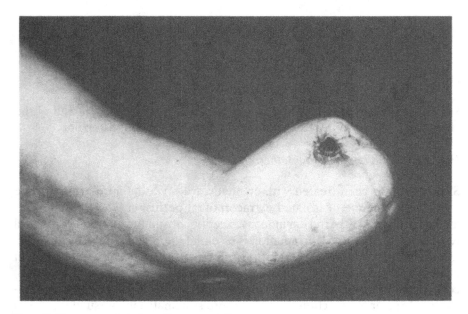

Figure 6. Recurrence in below elbow amputation stump.

Factors affecting the degree of disability are the extent of surgery and the sophistication of radiation technique. While most oncologists strive to conserve a functional limb and few patients wish otherwise, two studies [26, 27] that compared psychosocial outcome between such patients and amputees failed to demonstrate any advantage for the former group, as judged by the parameters measured.

Retroperitoneal sarcomas

Sarcomas of the retroperitoneum account for ~12% of all malignant soft tissue tumors [28]. The limitation to wide-field, radical-dose irradiation imposed by the abdominal viscera means that complete surgical extirpation is essential for long-term control and hence survival [29–31]. Bowel, kidney, and major vessels may need to be sacrificed in order to gain clear margins, though clearance will inevitably be narrow because of the local anatomy. Karakousis [32] has described an abdominoinguinal approach to the difficult tumor involving the lower retroperitoneum. For the upper retroperitoneum, free use should be made of the standard thoracoabdominal exposure. It has been suggested that postoperative irradiation may be of some benefit, especially when resection margins are unsatisfactory, and the use of intraoperative radiotherapy and brachytherapy warrants further investigation [33]. Adjuvant cytotoxic therapy has shown no advantage [30].

Omental flaps [34] and synthetic mesh [35] have been used after pelvic

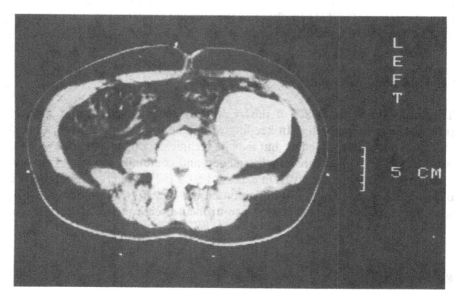

Figure 7. Computerized tomographic scan of abdomen: 500-ml Dow Corning mammary prosthesis inserted as spacer following excision of sarcoma arising from anterior surface of psoas.

exenteration to exclude small intestine from the pelvic cavity and thus avoid postoperative radiation damage to the bowel. Similar principles can be applied following surgery for sarcoma and, in two of the author's patients, a Dow Corning mammary prosthesis, supplemented by omentum in one, has been positioned as a spacer for this purpose (Fig. 7).

Sarcomas of the chest and abdominal wall

As with sarcomas at other sites, the key to successful local management is excision with clear margins [36, 37]. Surgical planning is greatly assisted by computerized tomography, which helps define the lateral extent of the tumor and indicates whether the pleura or peritoneum and the underlying viscera are involved.

Current reconstructive techniques allow uninhibited resection, and extensive, full-thickness defects can be readily managed [38]. Stabilization as well as cover are required to protect the viscera, prevent herniation and, in the case of the thoracic cage, to limit paradoxical movement. Patients undergoing major chest wall surgery often need postoperative respiratory support in the intensive care unit. For stabilization of most defects, one should consider the use of polypropylene mesh, which can be shaped as desired and is well tolerated by the tissues. Occasionally, muscle flaps alone are sufficient for this purpose. In the case of postirradiation sarcomas [39], it is important to introduce well-vascularized tissues into the repair, e.g., latissimus dorsi or rectus abdominis myocutaneous flaps, or the mobilized greater omentum [40]. Weinstein et al. [41] emphasized the value of the tensor fasciae latae flap in abdominal wall repair.

Sarcomas of the head and neck

The anatomical complexity of this region precludes description of surgical procedures at specific sites. In keeping with general principles, wide surgical clearance should be aimed at, but may be technically difficult to achieve. Adjuvant therapy is therefore usually needed and combined-modality management can yield 5-year survivals in excess of 50% [42]. The critical importance of local disease control in this difficult area was shown by Harmer et al. [43], who found that death was due to uncontrolled disease at the primary site in 65% of their patients.

References

1. Lindberg RL, Martin RG, Romsdahl MM, Barkley HT: Conservative surgery with postoperative radiotherapy in 300 adults with soft-tissue sarcomas. Cancer 47:2391–2397, 1981.

2. Collin C, Hadju SI, Godbolt J, Shiu MH, Hilaris BI, Brennan MF: Localized, operable soft tissue sarcoma of the lower extremity. Arch Surg 121:1425–1433, 1986.

3. Collin C, Hajdu SI, Godbold J, Friedrich C, Brennan MF: Localized operable soft tissue sarcoma of the upper extremity: presentation, management and factors affecting local recurrence in 108 patients. Ann Surg 205:331–339, 1986.

4. Abbatucci JS, Boulier N, De Ranieri J, Mandard AM, Tanguy A, Vernhes JC, Lozier JC, Busson A: Local control and survival in soft tissue sarcomas of the limbs, trunk walls and head and neck: a study of 113 cases. Int J Radiat Oncol Biol Phys 12:579–586, 1986.

5. Wood WC, Suit HD, Mankin HJ, Cohen AM, Proppe K: Radiation and conservative surgery in the treatment of soft tissue sarcoma. Am J Surg 147:537–541, 1984.

6. Rouesse JG, Friedman S, Sevin DM, Le Chevalier T, Spielmann ML, Contesso G, Sarrazin DM, Genin JR: Preoperative induction chemotherapy in the treatment of locally advanced soft tissue sarcomas. Cancer 60:296–300, 1987.

7. Muchmore JH, Carter RD, Krementz ET: Regional perfusion for malignant melanoma and soft tissue sarcoma: a review. Cancer Invest 3:129–143, 1985.

8. Eilber FR, Guilliano AE, Huth J, Mirra J, Morton DL: High-grade soft-tissue sarcomas of the extremity: UCLA experience with limb salvage. In: Primary chemotherapy in cancer medicine. New York: Alan R Liss, 1985, 59–74.

9. Enneking WF, Spanier SS, Malawer MM: The effect of anatomic setting on the results of surgical procedures for soft parts sarcoma of the thigh. Cancer 47:1005–1022, 1981.

10. Mankin HJ, Lange TA, Spanier SS: The hazards of biopsy in patients with primary bone and soft tissue tumours. J Bone Joint Surg [Am] 64:1121–1127, 1982.

11. Westbury G: Soft tissue sarcomas. In: Keen, G (ed): Operative Surgical Management. Bristol: Wright, 1987, pp 757–765.

12. Kissin MW, Fisher C, Carter RL, Horton LWL, Westbury G: Value of Tru-cut biopsy in the diagnosis of soft tissue tumours. Br J Surg 73:742–744, 1986.

13. Kissin MW, Fisher C, Webb AJ, Westbury G: Value of fine needle aspiration cytology in the diagnosis of soft tissue tumours: a preliminary study on the excised specimen. Br J Surg 74:479–480, 1987.

14. National Institutes of Health consensus development panel on limb-sparing treatment of adult soft tissue sarcomas and osteosarcomas. Cancer Treat Symp 3:1–5, 1985.

15. Cade S: Soft tissue tumours: their natural history and treatment. Proc R Soc Med 44:19–36, 1951.

16. Potter DA, Kinsella T, Glatstein E, Wesley R, White DE, Seipp CA, Chang AE, Lack EE, Costa J, Rosenberg SA: High-grade soft tissue sarcomas of the extremities. Cancer 58:190–205, 1986.

17. Enneking WF, McAuliffe JA: Adjunctive preoperative radiation therapy in the treatment of soft tissue sarcomas: a preliminary report. Cancer Treat Symp 3:37–42, 1985.

18. Bramwell VHC, Crowther D, Deakin DP, Swindell R, Harris M: Combined modality management of local and disseminated adult soft tissue sarcomas: a review of 257 cases seen over 10 years at the Christie Hospital and Holt Radium Institute, Manchester. Br J Cancer 51:301–318, 1985.

19. Suit HD, Mankin HJ, Schiller AL, Wood WC, Tepper JE, Gebhardt MC: Results of treatment of sarcoma of soft tissue by radiation and surgery at Massachusetts General Hospital. Cancer Treat Symp 3:43–47, 1985.

20. Lindberg R: Treatment of localised soft tissue sarcoma in adults at M.D. Anderson Hospital and Tumor Institute (1960–1981). Cancer Treat Symp 3:59–65, 1985.

21. Okunieff P, Suit HD, Proppe KH: Extremity preservation by combined modality treatment of sarcomas of the hand and wrist. Int J Radiat Oncol Biol Phys 12:1923–1929, 1986.

22. Suit HD, Mankin HJ, Wood WC, Proppe KH: Preoperative, intraoperative, and postoperative radiation in the treatment of primary soft tissue sarcoma. Cancer 55:2659–2667, 1985.

23. Arbeit JM, Hilaris BS, Brennan MF: Wound complications in the multimodality treatment of extremity and superficial truncal sarcomas. J Clin Oncol 5:480–488, 1987.

24. Lehti PM, Moseley HS, Janoff K, Stevens K, Fletcher WS: Improved survival for soft tissue sarcoma of the extremities by regional hyperthermic perfusion, local excision and radiation therapy. Surg Gynecol Obstet 162:149–152, 1986.
25. Lampert MH, Gerber LH, Glatstein E, Rosenberg SA, Danoff JV: Soft tissue sarcoma: functional outcome after wide local excision and radiation therapy. Arch Phys Med Rehabil 65:477–480, 1984.
26. Sugarbaker PH, Barofsky I, Rosenberg SA, Gianola FJ: Quality of life assessment of patients in extremity sarcoma clinical trials. Surgery 91:17–23, 1982.
27. Weddington WW, Blindt Segraves K, Simon MA: Psychological outcome of extremity sarcoma survivors undergoing amputation or limb salvage. J Clin Oncol 3:1393–1399, 1985.
28. Lawrence W, Donegan WL, Natarajan N, Mettlin C, Beart R, Winchester D: Adult soft tissue sarcomas: a pattern of care survey of the American College of Surgeons. Ann Surg 205:349–359, 1987.
29. McGrath PC, Neifeld JP, Lawrence W, DeMay RM, Kay S, Horsley, JS, Parker GA: Improved survival following complete excision of retroperitoneal sarcomas. Ann Surg 200: 200–204, 1984.
30. Glenn J, Sindelar WF, Kinsella T, Glatstein E, Tepper J, Costa J, Baker A, Sugarbaker P, Brennan MF, Seipp C, Wesley R, Young RC, Rosenberg SA: Results of multimodality therapy of resectable soft-tissue sarcomas of the retroperitoneum. Surgery 97:316–324, 1985.
31. Karakousis CP, Velez AF, Emrich LJ: Management of retroperitoneal sarcomas and patient survival. Am J Surg 150:376–380, 1985.
32. Karakousis CP: Utility of the abdominoinguinal incision in the resection of lower abdominal tumours. J Surg Oncol 26:176–182, 1984.
33. Harrison, LB, Gutierrez E, Fischer JJ: Retroperitoneal sarcomas: the Yale experience and a review of the literature. J Surg Oncol 32:159–164, 1986.
34. Jakowatz JG, Porudominsky D, Riihimaki DU, Kemeny M, Kokal WA, Braly PS, Terz JJ, Beatty JD: Complications of pelvic exenteration. Arch Surg 120:1261–1265, 1985.
35. Buchsbaum HJ, Christopherson W, Lifshitz S, Bernstein S: Vicryl mesh in pelvic floor reconstruction. Arch Surg 120:1389–1391, 1985.
36. Greager JA, Patel MK, Briele HA, Walker MJ, Wood DK, Das Gupta TK: Soft tissue sarcomas of the adult thoracic wall. Cancer 59:370–373, 1987.
37. Shiu MH, Flancbaum L, Hajdu SI, Fortner JG: Malignant soft-tissue tumors of the anterior abdominal wall. Arch Surg 115:152–155, 1980.
38. Pailolero PC, Arnold PG: Thoracic wall defects: surgical management of 205 consecutive patients. Mayo Clin Proc 61:557–563, 1986.
39. Souba WW, McKenna RJ, Meis J, Benjamin R, Raymond AK, Mountain CF: Radiation-induced sarcomas of the chest wall. Cancer 57:610–615, 1986.
40. Williams R, White H: The greater omentum: its applicability to cancer surgery and cancer therapy. Curr Probl Surg 23:818–828, 1986.
41. Weinstein LP, Kovachev D, Chaglassian T: Abdominal wall reconstruction. Scand J Plas Reconstr Surg 20:109–113, 1986.
42. Greager JA, Das Gupta TK: Adult head and neck soft-tissue sarcomas. Otolaryngol Clin North Am 19:565–571, 1986.
43. Harmer CL, Frampton M, Wiltshaw E: Role of radiotherapy and chemotherapy in management of soft tissue sarcomas. In: Bloom HJG, Hanham IWF, Shaw HJ (eds): Head and neck oncology. New York: Raven, 1987, pp 237–252.

5. The role for radiation therapy in the management of patients with sarcoma of soft tissue in 1988

Herman D. Suit

Over the past two decades, major changes have occured in the strategy of management of virtually all patients with sarcoma of soft tissue and bone. These changes have been primarily directed to combining less radical surgery with radiation and or chemotherapy so as to improve the cosmetic and functional quality of the local result and to increase disease-free survival rates. These combined-modality treatments have been tested clinically and substantial gains have been realized.

In this chapter, consideration is given to sarcomas of soft tissue other than rhabdomyosarcoma of pediatric patients. For sarcomas of soft tissue, the use of surgery alone for other than the small and low-grade lesions is now infrequent. Instead, moderate-dose radiation is combined with conservative surgery with impressive gains in cosmetic and functional results and apparently even lower local failure rates. This development is interesting because of the fact that, until the 1960s, sarcomas were classed as radiation resistant. The opinions expressed in major textbooks and the judgment of most clinicans working in this area were that radiation had no role to play in the management of patients with these tumors [1]. These opinions were based on the limited experience in the 1930s and 1940s with low-energy x-rays [250–300 kilovolts (peak)] and low total doses ($\approx 40–45$ Gy) as the sole treatment of patients with large sarcomas. However, radiation can be effective against *small* sarcomas when high radiation doses are employed [2–5].

In 1956, Puck and associates [6, 7] published the first radiation survival curves for mammalian cells. Their findings implied that there was a relatively narrow range in radiation sensitivity (as described in terms of values of the parameters D_0 and n) of cell lines derived from epithelial and mesenchymal tissues, normal and malignant. Accordingly, cells of sarcomas might not necessarily be of unusual radiation resistance. These considerations encouraged the testing of the then available supervoltage radiation against sarcomas of soft tissues. The experience in the 1960s was largely based on patients seen following relatively conservative surgical resections. That experience differed from the earlier work in two critically important aspects: (a) high radiation doses were employed (≈ 60 Gy), and (b) the number of tumor cells was greatly reduced as a consequence of prior resection of the grossly evident tumor

Pinedo, H.M., Verweij, J., eds. TREATMENT OF SOFT TISSUE SARCOMAS.
© Kluwer Academic Publishers, Boston. ISBN: 0-89838-391-9. All rights reserved.

mass. The results were indeed satisfactory with a local control rate of ~80% [8, 9], similar to that achieved by radical surgery. Comparable results have been obtained in many other centers; chemotherapy has also been employed in some of the series [10–15]. The impact has been a steep decline in the use of radical resection alone and/or amputation for patients with primary sarcoma of soft tissue. In addition, radiation has been employed in combination with amputation to reduce the likelihood of recurrence in the surgical stump when amputation is judged to be associated with a very close or nonexistent margins.

The current staging systems for sarcoma of soft tissue employ the histopathological grade of tumor as the principal determinant of stage. According to the revised staging system of the American Joint Commission for Cancer Staging and End Results Reporting (AJC) Stages I, II, and III are comprised of tumors of grades 1, 2, and 3, respectively [16]. Thus, the histopathologist's role is of critical importance in providing estimates of the prognosis for the individual patient. Further, we consider that the grade of tumor is an indicator of the extent of local infiltration and not only the probability of distant metastasis. Namely, the margins for the radiation treatment volume or the surgical resection are larger for G3 than G1 sarcomas.

Regional lymph node involvement in patients with sarcoma of soft tissue is a function of grade and size of tumor. A recent review of the world literature showed that the overall incidence of involvement of regional lymph nodes at diagnosis or as the first site of metastatic disease was 3.9% [17]. In the Massachusetts General Hospital series, there was no regional node involvement in patients with Grade I disease. Virtually all of the regional node involvement occurred in patients with Grade III sarcomas. Of these, essentially all occurred in patients whose Grade III sarcoma was >5 cm [17].

Rationale for combining radiation and surgery

The basic concept for combining radiation and surgery is quite simple. Namely, the surgical procedure was extended from simple excision (with an associated local failure rate of 70%–90%) to radical resection (local failure rate of 10%–20%) in order to remove the grossly normal tissue that was involved on a microscopic basis. Moderate doses of radiation are effective in eradication of the small number of tumor cells that have infiltrated beyond the gross lesion. Thus, by combining well-tolerated doses of radiation with conservative surgery, local control is achieved with minimal loss of grossly uninvolved tissue [13].

Todoroki and Suit [18] have investigated the combination of radiation and surgery using early generation isotransplants of a spontaneous fibrosarcoma (FSaII) growing in the leg of the syngeneic C3H mouse as the model system. Radiation followed by conservative excision sharply reduced the dose required to eradicate the fibrosarcoma; the dose was only slightly furhter reduced by radical resection. The "clinical efficacy" as measured by the degree of leg shortening for a given tumor control probability was higher for radiation combined with limited than with radical resection.

Results of combining radiation and surgery

Table 1 shows the current status and 5-year actuarial results in 258 consecutive patients treated at the Massachusetts General Hospital by conservative surgery and radiation according to AJC stage over the period of 1971 to June 1986. There have been 26 local failures and 60 patients have developed distant metastasis with local control. Further, 17 patients have died of intercurrent disease. The overall actuarial local control and survival rates at 5 years were 88% and 74%, respectively [19]. These results compare favorably with those obtained by radical surgry alone when performed by surgeons specializing in the management of patients with sarcomas [20, 21]. The survival figures are relatively good for lesions <5 cm and decline only slightly with grade, i.e., 100%, 93%, and 83% for Grades I, III, and III lesions, respectively. For the large lesions, however, survival decreased rapidly with tumor grade, namely, 96%, 65%, and 46% for Grades I, II, and III, respectively. In Table 2, the 5-year actuarial local control results are presented according to size of the sarcoma for patients treated with radiation given preoperatively or postoperatively. For the postoperative treatments, patients received doses of $\approx 64-66$ Gy. The dose for patients given radiation preoperatively has been 50–56 Gy followed by a boost dose of 10–15 Gy given intraoperatively by brachytherapy or postoperatively by external beam techniques with the radiation directed to the tumor bed as defined by surgical clips. Currently, the preoperative radiation dose is 50 Gy if given on a Q.D.

Table 1. Current status and 5-year actuarial results in 258 patients treated at Massachusetts General Hospital by conservative surgery and radiation according to stage [19]

Stages	No. of patients	NED	LF ± DM	DM	ID	5-year actuarial (%)	
						Local control	Survival
IA	17	16	—		1	100	100
B	30	24	2	2	2	93	96
IIA	40	28	4	5	3	88	93
B	66	33	8	22	3	85	65
IIIA	33	26	2	2	3	93	88
B	69	25	10	29	5	79	46
IVA	3	3	—	—		100	100
Total	258	155	26	60	17	88	74

NED, no evident disease; LF, local failure; DM, distant metastasis; and ID, dead of intercurrent disease.

Table 2. Five-year actuarial local control and survival results according to size [19]

Size (mm)	Postoperative			Preoperative		
	No. of patients	LC (%)	Survival (%)	No. of patients	LC (%)	Survival (%)
≤25	21	86	94	9	100	100
26–49	44	92	90	11	91	90
50–100	57	86	67	48	92	75
101–150	12	91	82	21	100	48
151–200	7	54	71	18	70	47
>200	3	67	67	7	100	43
Total	144	86	79	114	91	67

LC, local control.

Table 3. Five-year actuarial local control and survival results among 258 patients treated by radiation and surgery according to time period of treatment [19]

Time period	Postoperative			Preoperative		
	No. of patients	LC (%)	Survival (%)	No. of patients	LC (%)	Survival (%)
1971–75	33	81	79	4	100	25
1976–80	48	83.7	80	28	77	61
1980–86	63	92	80	82	97	73
Total	144			114		

LC, local control.

or 45 Gy if given on a B.I.D. basis, using 1.8 Gy per fraction. The actuarial local control results at 5 years were 86% and 91% for the postoperatively and preoperatively treated groups, respectively. Local control results were equivalent or higher in the preoperative group at all tumor size categories. An advantage of preoperative radiation appears to obtain for the patients with large sarcomas, viz., ≥10 cm [19]. Local control and survival results have improved with time. In the most recent period (Table 3), 1980–1986, local control rates were 92% and 97% for the postoperative and the preoperative group (based on 63 and 82 patients), respectively. Similarly, disease-free survival rates have been higher. Interestingly, this has occurred during a period when the proportion of patients being treated by radiation alone has declined from 33% to something less now than 10%. Very few patients are currently being judged to be inoperable when radiation is given preoperatively. The lower survival rates in the preoperative series reflect the larger tumors in that series.

There are other effective strategies for the conservative treatment of primary sarcomas of soft tissue. For example, Eilber and associates at UCLA have employed intra-arterial infusion of adriamycin combined with radiation given in fractions of 3.5 Gy [15, 22] (see also chapter 8). In their clinic, the radiation dose initially was 10 × 3.5 Gy; because of excessive treatment-related morbidity, this was reduced to 5 × 3.5 Gy. Recently, the dose has been raised to 8 × 3.5 Gy because of higher local failure rates. They currently achieve local control rates of 90%–95%.

Functional status

These efforts to preserve anatomy and function have realized worthwhile successes. For example, only five of our patients with extremity sarcomas have had an amputation. Further, ~75%–80% have retained good function, i.e., they do not need support devices and are free of pain. In the other 20%–25%, patients require the use of a cane or some support device, or the use of pressure stocking to regulate edema. Pain is an uncommon problem among these patients. In the patients treated preoperatively, there may be delay in wound healing, especially among older and obese patients with large sarcomas. This is particularly a problem in patients whose sarcoma is located in the proximal thigh. Fortunately, the wounds do heal even though some hospital care may be required. Special efforts directed to facilitate the wound healing include, for example, the use of flaps where there is to be any tension in the wound closure, the use of transposed muscle to help reduce the defect produced by the removal of a large tumor mass, and monitoring of the wound for residual fluid before removal of drainage tubes.

Specific techniques

Proton beam radiation therapy

We have now treated 12 patients with sarcoma of the paraspinal tissues. Of these 12, four had gross disease and only two of these have had local control. In the eight patients irradiated for positive margins, there have been no local failures. Because of the ability to contour the dose distribution in depth by varying the energy of the protons coming in along each voxel, we have given only small doses to the spinal cord. As expected, there has been no instance of damage to the spinal cord although the dose to the tumor bed was carried to full levels, i.e., 64–66 Gy (Austin-Seymour et al., unpublished data, 1988).

Further, three patients whose sarcoma overlay the hip joint had part of their treatment by an anterior proton beam. The treatment was planned so that the protons penetrated to the joint capsule. Joint function has been good; fibrosis of the overlying subcutaneous tissue has been significant in the three patients.

Fast neutron beam radiation therapy

Experience is being acquired in several centers with fast neutron beam radiation therapy for sarcomas of soft tissue; some of this is interpreted as encouraging [23–25]. The published reports do not describe outcomes of treatment for tumors stratified according to size and grade. Results of a phase III clinical trial of fast neutron beam vs photon beam (alone or combined with surgery) are not yet available. From several case reports, there clearly have been some impressive complete responses of sarcomas of substantial proportions. Hopefully, a clear gain for fast neutrons will be demonstrated. However, there is apparently an important problem with the fast neutron therapy, viz., evidently a marked increase in late damage in normal tissue [26].

Negative pion therapy

The report from the Swiss Institute for Nuclear studies (SIN) [27] on their experience with pion beam treatment of patients with retroperitoneal sarcoma is highly encouraging. Evidently good results against this formidable group of tumors are being realized.

Hyperthermia

There would appear to be a real potential for combining hyperthermia with radiation in the treatment of the infrequent inoperable sarcoma. The interest in hyperthermia is that the age response functions for hyperthermic and radiation cell killing are complementary. Further, because of the poor vascular supply and blood perfusion characteristics, the large sarcoma should experience a higher temperature than the surrounding normal tissues. There are very few data on the experience with hyperthermia in the treatment of this category of tumors at present.

Specific tumors

Desmoids and aggressive fibromatosis

One of the developments over the past decade or so has been the realization that desmoid tumors (aggressive fibromatosis) can be controlled in a high proportion of cases by radiation alone, viz., ≈ 60 Gy. These lesions should be resected where this is feasible. Not infrequently, desmoid tumors arise in anatomic sites that preclude effective surgery or result in major morbidity. In those circumstances, radiation may be considered as an alternate, with an expected long-term local control rate of $\approx 80\%$ [28–32]. The indications for radiation in patients with desmoids are not straightforward. For example, a patient who has had resection of a primary desmoid tumor, but with positive margins, is not a definite candidate for postoperative radiation. In our institution, we have followed 16 patients with positive margins at resection of their *primary* tumor (Miralbell and Suit, unpublished data, 1988); $\sim 35\%-40\%$ of these patients ultimately show locally recurrent tumor, i.e., $\simeq 60\%$ do not recur. This is supported by the report by Reitmao et al. [33] that 17% of their patients who had an incomplete removal ultimately developed local recurrence. Because of the high success of radiation treatment of desmoid tumors and absence of risk for distant metastasis, we now defer treatment unless the lesion was in a site where recurrence would be quite difficult to manage. At our institution, all patients who had incomplete removal for a *recurrent* desmoid are subjected to additional surgery or radiation. All patients whose primary or recurrent lesions are not operable are accepted for radiation treatment. There are several provocative reports of occasional success in the treatment of desmoid tumors by means of antiestrogens and nonsteroid anti-inflammatory drugs [34, 35].

Dermatofibrosarcoma protuberans

A brief comment here is in order regarding the potential role of radiation treatment for dermatofibrosarcoma protuberans. Marks and Suit (1988, unpublished) have reviewed the experience at the Massachusetts General Hospital in the treatment of patients with dermatofibrosarcoma protuberans with radiation. Eight patients have been treated. The observation period is 1–5 years. Five patients were treated by radiation and surgery (four postoperative for incomplete margins, and one by preoperative radiation and then resection). Three patients were treated by radiation alone. All eight patients have no evidence of disease. This is clearly a small series and the observation is brief. The data do, however, indicate that, in the occasional patient with dermatofibrosarcoma protuberans whose lesion is nonresectable or has positive margins, radiation can be considered as an appropriate modality.

Clinical research problems relating to the combination of radiation and surgery

These include: (1) Under what circumstance should the radiation be given before surgery? (2) How high should the radiation dose be? (3) What is the extent of the involvement of tissue by subclinical disease as a function of grade, size, and site, i.e., what is the magnitude of the target volume for the subclinical disease? (4) Should the radiation dose he given on a Q.D. or a B.I.D. basis for high-grade sarcomas? (5) Should the dose per fraction be in the range of 1.8–2.0 Gy or a very small dose per fraction, $\simeq 1.0-1.2$ Gy? (6) To what extent can the scope of the surgery be reduced? Namely, is a margin of grossly normal tissue around the gross tumor necessary? This is an important question since the margins are usually quite close in at least one dimension. (7)

How should the radiation treatment in terms of dose per fraction, total dose, and timing be modified if combined with chemotherapy? (8) What roles do high linear-energy-transfer radiation and hyperthermia have in management of this group of patients?

Conclusion

In the last decade, we have witnessed a shift in the applicability of radiotherapy in the treatment of soft tissue sarcomas. The usefulness of combining surgery with postoperative radiation is clear to all investigators. The use of pre- and postoperative radiation and new techniques have generated very interesting preliminary data indicating that the previous belief that soft tissue sarcomas are absolutely radioresistant will have to be revised.

Acknowledgments

The author is pleased to acknowledge the contributions of colleagues in surgery, medicine, pathology, and radiology in the management of these patients, particularly Drs. H. Mankin, W. Wood, A. Rosenberg, A. Schiller, D. Rosenthal, M. Gebhardt, and J. Tepper. The excellent work of Claire Hunt in preparation of the manuscript of this chapter is greatly appreciated.

References

1. Paterson R: The treatment of malignant disease by radium and x-rays. London: Edward Arnold, 1953.
2. Cade S: Soft tissue tumours: their natural history and treatment. Section of Surgery. President's address. Proc R Soc Med 44:19–36, 1951.
3. McNeer GP, et al.: Effectiveness of radiation therapy in management of sarcoma of soft somatic tissues. Cancer 22:391–397, 1968.
4. Windeyer B, Dische S, Mansfield CM: The place of radiotherapy in the management of fibrosarcoma of the soft tissues. Clin Radiol 17:32–40, 1966.
5. Tepper JE, Suit HD: Radiation therapy alone for sarcoma of soft tissue. Cancer 56:475–479, 1985.
6. Puck TT, Marcus PI: Action of x-rays on mammalian cells. J Exp Med 105:653–666, 1956.
7. Puck TT, Morkovin D, Marcus PI, Cieciura SJ: Action of x-rays on mammalian cells. II. Survival curves of cells from normal human tissues. J Exp Med 106:485–500, 1957.
8. Suit HD, Russell WO, Martin RG: Management of patients with sarcoma of soft tissue in an extremity. Cancer 31:1247–1255, 1973.
9. Suit HD, Russell WO, Martin RG: Sarcoma of soft tissue: clinical and histopathologic parameters and response to treatment. Cancer 35:1478–1483, 1975.
10. Collins JE, Paine CH, Ellis F: Treatment of connective tissue sarcomas by local excision followed by radioactive implant. Clin Radiol 27:39–41, 1976.
11. Rosenberg SA, et al.: Prospective randomised evaluation of the role of limb sparing surgery, radiation therapy and adjuvant chemotherapy in the treatment of adult soft tissue sarcomas. Surgery 84:62–69, 1978.

12. Lindberg RD: Conservative surgery and post-operative radiotherapy in 300 adults with soft-tissue sarcomas. Cancer 47:2391–2397, 1981.
13. Suit HD, Mankin HJ, Wood WC, Proppe KH: Radiation and surgery in the treatment of primary sarcoma of soft tissue: pre-operative, intra-operative and post-operative. Cancer 55: 2659–2667, 1985.
14. Lehti PM et al.: Improved survival for soft tissue sarcoma of the extremities by regional hyperthermic perfusion, local excision and radiation therapy. Surg Gynecol Obstet 162: 149–152, 1986.
15. Eilber FR, Giuliano A, Huth J, Mirra J, Rosen G, Morton D: Neoadjuvant chemotherapy, radiation, and limited surgery for high grade soft tissue sarcoma of the extremity. In: Recent Concepts in Sarcoma Treatment (Proceedings of the Internat Symp on Sarcomas, Florida, 1987). Eds., JR Ryan, LH Baker, Kluwer Academic Pub., Dordrecht, the Netherlands, 1988, pp 115–122.
16. TNM Classification of Malignant Tumours. Edition 4. International Union against Cancer. P Hermanck and LH Sobin, eds. Springerverlag, 1988.
17. Mazeron JJ, Suit HD: Lymph nodes as sites of metastasis from sarcomas of soft tissue. Cancer 60:1800–1808, 1987.
18. Todoroki T, Suit HD: Therapeutic advantage in pre-operative single dose radiation combined with conservative and radical surgery in different size murine fibrosarcomas. J Surg Oncol 29:207–215, 1985.
19. Suit HD, Mankin HJ, Willett CG, Gebhardt MC, Wood WC, Skates S: Limited surgery and external irradiation in soft tissue sarcomas. In: Recent Concepts in Sarcoma Treatment (Proceedings of the Internat Symp on Sarcomas, Tarpon Springs, Florida, 1987). Eds., JR Ryan, LH Baker, Kluwer Academic Pub., Dordrecht, the Netherlands, 1988, pp 94–103.
20. Enneking WF, Spanier SS, Malawar MD: The effect of anatomic setting on the results of surgical procedures for soft parts sarcoma of the thigh. Cancer 47:1005, 1981.
21. Markhede G, Angervall L, Stener B: A multivariate analysis of the prognosis after surgical treatment of malignant soft tissue tumors. Cancer 40:1721–1733, 1982.
22. Eilber FR, et al.: High grade soft tissue sarcomas of the extremity: UCLA experience with limb salvage. Prog Clin Biol Res 201:59–74, 1985.
23. Franke HD, Schmidt R: Clinical results after therapy with fast neutrons (DT, 14 MeV) since 1976 in Hamburg-Eppendorf. In: Karcher KH (ed) Progress in radio-oncology, vol 3: Proceedings of the third meeting on progress in radio-oncology, Vienna, 1986. Vienna: Internat Club of Radio-Oncology, 1987, pp 164–174.
24. Schmitt G, Scherer E, von Essen CF: Neutron and neutron boost irradiation of soft tissue sarcomas. Strahlentherapie 161:784–786, 1985.
25. Laramore G, Griffeth JT, Boespflug M, Pelton JG, Griffin TW, Griffin BR, Russell AJ, Koh W: Fast neutron radiotherapy for sarcoma of soft tissue, bone, and cartilage. Am J Clin Oncol (in press).
26. Duncan W, Arnott SJ, Jack WJL: The Edinburgh experience of treating sarcomas of soft tissues and bone with neutron irradiation. Clin Radiol 37:317–320, 1986.
27. Schmitt G, von Essen CF, Griener R, Blattmann H: Review of the SIN and Los Alamos Pion Trials. Radiat Res 104:S-272–S-278, 1985.
28. Kiel K, Suit HD: Radiation therapy in the treatment of aggressive fibromatoses (desmoid tumors). Cancer 54:2051–2055, 1984.
29. Benninghoff D, Robbins R: The nature and treatment of desmoid tumors. AJR 91:132–137, 1964.
30. Leibel SA, Wara WM, Hill DR, et al.: Desmoid tumors: local control and patterns of relapse following radiation therapy. Int J Radiat Oncol Biol Phys 9:1167–1171, 1983.
31. Greenberg HM, Goebel R, Weichselbaum RR, Greenberger JS, Chaffey JT, Cassady JR: Radiation therapy in the treatment of aggressive fibromatosis. Int J Radiat Oncol Biol Phys 7:305–310, 1981.
32. Keus R, Bartelink H: The role of radiotherapy in the treatment of desmoid tumours. Radiother Oncol 7:1–5, 1986.

33. Reitamo JJ, Scheinin TM, Hayry P: The desmoid syndrome: new aspects in the cause, pathogenesis and treatment of the desmoid tumor. Am J Surg 151:230–237, 1986.
34. Lim CL, Walker MJ, Mehta RR, Das Gupta TK: Estrogen and antigestrogen binding sites in desmoid tumors. Europ J Cancer and Clinic Oncol 22(5):583–587.
35. Waddell WR, Gerner RE, Reich MP: Nonsteroid antiinflammatory drugs and tamoxifen for desmoid tumors and carcinoma of the stomach. J Surg Oncol 22:197–211, 1983.

6. Chemotherapy in advanced soft tissue sarcomas

Jaap Verweij, Cees J. van Groeningen, and Herbert M. Pinedo

With local recurrence rates of 40%–80% [1] and most of these relapses occurring within 3 years [2], soft tissue sarcomas have always been a difficult tumor type for adequate local treatment. Although sophisticated surgical techniques and the addition of postoperative high-dose radiotherapy have considerably reduced the number of local recurrences in extremity lesions [2–5], the inability to apply the necessary high doses of irradiation precluded a decrease in local recurrence in truncal lesions by using the combination of surgery and radiotherapy. Besides, soft tissue sarcomas metastasize by (apparently early) hematogeneous spreading, most frequently to the lungs, which can only partly be prevented by optimal local control of the primary tumor. Therefore, distant metastases still occur in a considerable number of patients, for whom systemic treatment with chemotherapy will be considered.

This chapter summarizes previous achievements in the chemotherapy of advanced soft tissue sarcomas and discusses in detail some new developments and future topics.

Single-agent chemotherapy (Table 1)

Doxorubicin

The first drug identified as active single agent in the treatment of adult soft tissue sarcomas was doxorubicin (DX) [6], which, after this first report, has now been studied in almost 1200 patients [7, 8], yielding an overall response rate of 22% in nonpretreated patients, while preliminary data from a study by the European Organisation on Treatment and Research of Cancer (EORTC) also suggest activity of the drug in pretreated patients. A dose–response relationship has been established for DX, with doses of 60 mg/m^2 or more producing higher response rates than doses of 50 mg/m^2 or less [1, 9], when the drug is given every 3–4 weeks. The intermittent high-dose treatment schedule was generally assumed to be the most effective, but limited possibilities of combining DX with other myelosuppressive drugs and introduced the problem of cardiotoxicity. These limitations have stimulated studies on alterna-

Pinedo, H.M., Verweij, J., eds. TREATMENT OF SOFT TISSUE SARCOMAS.

Table 1. Active single agents

Drug	Previous chemotherapy	No. of patients	Response rate (%) Overall	Range	Ref.
Doxorubicin	No	1192	22	15–30	7, 8
DTIC	Yes	95	17	17–17	14, 15
Ifosfamide	No	93	24	23–25	20, 21
	Yes	117	36	7–65	16–21

tive schedules of DX administration, as well as research on less cardiotoxic anthracycline analogs.

Although previous studies suggested that weekly DX administration was equally as myelotoxic as one administration of DX every 3 weeks [10, 11], the recently reported Eastern Cooperative Oncology Group (ECOG) study randomizing DX 15 mg/m^2 weekly after an initial loading course, with DX 70 mg/m^2 every 3 weeks and with DX–DTIC (dacarbazine) [8], strongly indicates the opposite. The weekly DX administration resulted in more stomatitis (not significant) and less hematologic toxicity ($p > 0.05$) than did one administration of DX every 3 weeks. The weekly DX administration was as active (16% responses) as the administration of DX once every 3 weeks (18% responses), but this is a disappointing response rate for both.

One reason that the majority of soft tissue sarcoma patients do not respond to anthracyclines may be an overexpression of P-glycoprotein, as suggested by Gerlach et al. [12]. P-glycoprotein is a cell-surface glycoprotein involved in the active cellular outward transport of a.o. anthracyclines, and is overexpressed in association with the multidrug-resistant (MDR) phenotype. In six of 25 sarcoma patients, this MDR phenotype was found. Another alternative DX administration may be continuous infusion, which is thought to be less cardiotoxic [13]. However, its single-agent activity rate is unknown due to the absence of a phase II study.

The reasons for evaluating DX analogs in soft tissue sarcomas are obvious. Presently, DX is the most active single agent in this disease, while DX analogs are considered to have a more favorable therapeutic index as compared with the parent drug, mainly because of the expression of lesser degrees of myelosuppression and cardiac toxicity. The results of recently performed clinical trials with DX analogs and mitoxantrone are summarized in Table 2. Studies containing adequate numbers of patients are as yet limited. The EORTC Soft Tissue and Bone Sarcoma Group evaluated two DX analogs, carminomycin and epirubicin, respectively. Both drugs were compared in a randomized phase II trial with the parent drug, DX. Importantly, both studies were performed in patients without previous chemotherapy, which offered the new drugs an optimal chance to express significant antitumor activity.

Carminomycin [14] was shown to be inactive, while epirubicin [15] had

Table 2. Activity of doxorubicin analogs and mitoxantrone in advanced soft tissue sarcoma

Drug	No. of evaluable patients	No. of responders			Response rate (%)	Ref.
		CR	PR	Total		
Epirubicin	21 (20)	0	0	0	0	16
Epirubicin	84	4	11	15	18	15
vs						
doxorubicin	83	6	15	21	25	
Carminomycin	33	0	1	1	3	14
vs						
doxorubicin	38	1	10	11	29	
Aclarubicin	23	0	1	1	4	17
Idarubicin	35 (24)	1	1	2	6	19
Esorubicin	20 (1)	0	1	1	5	18
Mitoxantrone	46 (33)	0	0	0	0	20
Mitoxantrone	61 (61)	0	1	1	1.5	21

CR, complete remission; PR, partial remission; and ( ), number of patients with prior chemotherapy.

antitumor activity comparable to that of DX. The response rate (25%) to DX was slightly better than the response rate (18%) to epirubicin, but this difference was statistically not significant. On the other hand, toxicity of epirubicin was significantly less than that of DX, especially with respect to myelosuppression. These observations might be due to the fact that equimolar doses of both drugs were used. When doses of both drugs were used producing equal myelosuppression, it would not be surprising when epirubicin and DX were fully comparable in the treatment of soft tissue sarcoma, both with respect to efficacy and toxicity. However, a trial taking this into account has not been performed as yet. The only other study on epirubicin [16] was done in patients with prior chemotherapy, mainly consisting of DX-containing regimens. Not surprising, no responses were obtained. It seems highly unlikely that a significant number of DX-resistant patients will respond to subsequent treatment with epirubicin, due to cross resistance between epirubicin and DX. The occasional observation that cross resistance between both drugs may not be complete, as was suggested in the EORTC study [15], does not justify the use of epirubicin after resistance to the parent drug. The other DX analogs have been investigated to only a limited extent. Aclarubicin [17] and esorubicin [18] seem to have been evaluated in an adequate number of non-pretreated patients to conclude that both drugs are inactive in advanced soft tissue sarcoma. However, idarubicin [19] has mainly been studied in patients resistant to DX. Thus, a definite conclusion as to the efficacy of idarubicin is presently not possible.

Mitoxantrone, an anthraquinone derivative structurally related to DX, at present has been studied mainly in DX-resistant patients [20, 21], with minimal to absent antitumor activity. However, its value in nonpretreated patients is not known.

DTIC

The second drug with single-agent activity is DTIC. The first phase II study on this drug resulted in a 17% response rate in 53 patients [22]. Based on this single report, the drug was incorporated into combination chemotherapy. Only recently could the data be confirmed by a phase II study conducted by the EORTC Soft Tissue and Bone Sarcoma Group. Using DTIC at a dose of 1.2 g/m^2 by short-term infusion every 3 weeks, they achieved one complete and six partial remissions in 42 evaluable patients [23], with relatively limited toxicity.

Ifosfamide

The third active drug in the treatment of soft tissue sarcomas is ifosfamide (IFOS). Although the initially reported response rate of 65% [24] has never been confirmed, the compilation of all presently available reports indicates that the drug has activity comparable to that of DX (Table 1) [25–29]. Using the drug in a daily ×3–5 schedule appears to result in similar response rates as using the 24-h infusion once every 3 weeks. The optimal total dose of IFOS to be administered is 5 g/m^2. In pretreated patients, the overall response rate was 36% [24–29], while it was 24% in nonpretreated patients [28, 29], a difference mainly caused by the inclusion of the never-confirmed initial data in pretreated patients. The results of the two studies in nonpretreated patients are practically identical and offer a firm base for the conclusion that this drug has activity in the treatment of soft tissue sarcomas. On the other hand, the results obtained in nonpretreated patients clearly indicate that a truly active drug in soft tissue sarcomas will also be discovered by phase II studies in pretreated patients, a conclusion confirmed by the recent EORTC DTIC data [23]. Based on all IFOS studies, no single histological subtype has shown a preferential sensitivity for the drug, although it is interesting that four of eight patients with mixed mesodermal sarcomas, included in the EORTC study, responded [29].

Cyclophosphamide

Without the availability of single-agent data, cyclophosphamide has previously been incorporated into combination chemotherapy regimens. One of the important findings of the EORTC study randomizing IFOS versus cyclophosphamide was that cyclophosphamide cannot be considered to be a drug with interesting activity [29]. Even using a high dose of 1.5 g/m^2, the EORTC Soft Tissue and Bone Sarcoma Group achieved an overall response rate of only 8%: 13% for 38 nonpretreated patients and 0% for 29 pretreated patients.

Mixed mesodermal sarcoma may be the only histological subtype for which this cannot be concluded, because two of five patients did respond [29]. However, IFOS achieved similar results in this tumor type [29].

Other phase II studies

A variety of established and new antineoplastic agents have recently been studied in advanced soft tissue sarcoma. The results of the recently performed phase II studies on these drugs are summarized in Table 3. Of course, almost all of the patients in these trials had been pretreated with standard chemotherapy regimens. With one exception, disappointingly low response rates ranging from 0 to 6% were achieved in all of these studies. As a consequence, these drugs, inactive in pretreated patients, do not warrant testing up front. CDDP (cisplatin) is the only exception among the drugs listed in Table 3.

In a study by Sordillo et al. [38] of 26 nonpretreated patients, CDDP at a conventional dose of 120 mg/m^2 every 3–4 weeks did not show significant antitumor activity with a response rate of only 4%, confirming previous reports. In contrast, a study conducted by the Southwest Oncology Group (SWOG) [39] yielded a remarkable response rate of 24%. In this study, CDDP was used at a high dose of 40 mg/m^2 on 5 consecutive days, every 4 weeks. Moreover, all patients were heavily pretreated, while one patient had failed on a standard-dose CDDP regimen. Obviously, these data have to be confirmed by others before meaningful conclusions can be drawn, while the

Table 3. Activity of various established and new drugs in advanced soft tissue sarcoma

Drug	No. of evaluable patients	No. of responders			Response rate (%)	Ref.
		CR	PR	Total		
Methyl-GAG	18 (18)	0	0	0	0	30
Piperazinedione	19 (18)	0	1	1	5	31
Bleomycin	32 (32)	0	0	0	0	32
Chlorozotocin	37 (37)	0	1	1	3	32
MGBG	36 (36)	0	1	1	3	32
Bruceantin	34 (34)	0	0	0	0	32
Diaziquone	31 (31)	0	0	0	0	33
Bisantrene	17 (17)	0	0	0	0	34
Mitomycin C	16 (12)	0	1	1	6	35
Homoharringtonine	16 (16)	0	0	0	0	36
Cisplatin	19 (19)	1	0	1	5	37
Cisplatin	26 (0)	0	1	1	4	38
Cisplatin (high-dose)	17 (17)	0	4	4	24	39
TGU	19 (19)	0	0	0	0	40
VP-16	26 (24)	0	1	1	4	41
Fludarabine	20 (20)	0	0	0	0	42

CR, complete remission; PR, partial remission; and ( ), number of patients with prior chemotherapy.

Table 4. Activity of single-agent cisplatin in advanced mixed mesodermal sarcoma of the uterus

Dose/schedule	No. of evaluable patients	No. of responders			Response rate (%)	Ref.
		CR	PR	Total		
50 mg/m^2 i.v. q 3 weeks	28 (25)	2	3	5	18	45
75–100 mg/m^2 i.v. q 4 weeks	18 (7)	1	4	5	28	46

CR, complete remission; PR, partial remission; and ( ), number of patients with prior chemotherapy.

toxicity of such an approach also has to be taken into account. In contrast to other tumor types, data on biological response modifiers in the treatment of soft tissue sarcomas are very sparse.

In the recent literature, only two studies on interferon have been reported. In the first study [43], beta-interferon was evaluated in 20 patients, of whom 15 had received previous chemotherapy. One partial response was observed in a patient with fibrosarcoma. Gamma-interferon was studied by Edmonson et al. [44] in 16 patients with advanced soft tissue sarcomas; 14 patients had received prior chemotherapy. No objective responses were obtained. As for most other tumor types in advanced stages, interferons appear to be of little, if any, benefit to soft tissue sarcoma patients. The role of other biological response modifiers has presently not been tested in soft tissue sarcoma.

In contrast to the other types of soft tissue sarcoma, mixed mesodermal sarcoma of the uterus is sensitive to CDDP as was recently reported by Thigpen et al. [45] and Gershenson et al. [46] (Table 4). Of note, there were also responders among patients with prior chemotherapy. The relative insensitivity of mixed mesodermal sarcomas of the uterus to DX further distinguishes this disease from other soft tissue sarcomas as was recently reported by Morrow et al. [47].

VP-16 (etoposide) single-agent therapy has also recently been evaluated in this disease with a negative outcome [48]. In this study, 31 patients, 29 of whom had received previous chemotherapy, were treated with VP-16 at a dose of 100 mg/m^2 on days 1, 3, and 5, every 4 weeks. Only two patients experienced a short-term partial response.

In conclusion, in recent years, except for IFOS, no new antineoplastic agents or other treatment modalities have been developed for advanced soft tissue sarcomas. It is unlikely that epirubicin has a better therapeutic index as compared with DX in this disease, while the other DX analogs are probably inferior to the parent drug. Mitoxantrone has still to be evaluated in adequate numbers of nonpretreated patients. Definite results of high-dose CDDP should be awaited, as a preliminary report was promising. In mixed mesodermal sarcoma of the uterus, CDDP has shown definite activity, so incorporation of this drug into combination chemotherapy should be evaluated.

Combination chemotherapy

After having noted efficacy in preliminary reports on DX and DTIC single-agent treatment, and based upon suggested synergism in preclinical studies, the SWOG initiated a study, utilizing DX 60 mg/m^2 on day 1 and DTIC 250 mg/m^2/day on days 1–5, repeated every 3 weeks. This regimen is known as ADIC [Adriamycin (doxorubicin)–DTIC] [49]. Because of an initial responses rate of 42%, ADIC has also been studied by other groups, and recently interesting results using this combination have been published.

The ECOG has performed a randomized trial comparing DX 70 mg/m^2 i.v. bolus on day 1 every 3 weeks, with DX 20 mg/m^2 i.v. bolus on days 1, 2, and 3, and 15 mg/m^2 i.v. bolus on day 8 and weekly thereafter; and with DX 60 mg/m^2 i.v. bolus on day 1 plus DTIC 250 mg/m^2/day on days 1–5 repeated every 3 weeks [8]. This trial thus questioned the influence of the dosing schedule of DX and the value of the addition of DTIC. Regarding activity, the single-agent DX regimens resulted in comparable response rates (18% and 16%, respectively), while the addition of DTIC significantly ($p < 0.02$) increased the response rate to 30%, mainly by increasing the number of partial remissions. Unfortunately, the higher response rate of the combination was not reflected in an increased overall survival.

Although the combination was more toxic than the single-agent DX treatments, especially regarding gastrointestinal toxicity, this did not result in a lower treatment compliance, indicating that the combination side effects in general appear tolerable.

The Gynecologic Oncology Group (GOG) performed a quite similar trial in uterine sarcomas [50], comparing DX 60 mg/m^2 on day 1 every 3 weeks with the same dose of DX plus DTIC 250 mg/m^2/day on days 1–5 every 3 weeks. A response was achieved in 13 (16%) of 80 DX-treated patients and in 16 (24%) of 66 ADIC-treated patients. This difference in response rate is not significant in this subset of patients.

Two other randomized trials also questioned the value of the addition of other drugs to DX. The ECOG previously studied DX 70 mg/m^2 every 3 weeks, versus DX 50 mg/m^2 plus cyclophosphamide (CTX, or Cytoxan) 750 mg/m^2 plus vincristine (VCR) 1.4 mg/m^2 all by i.v. bolus on day 1 every 3 weeks, versus CTX 750 mg/m^2 plus VCR 1.4 mg/m^2 plus actinomycin-D (DACT, or dactinomycin) 0.4 mg/m^2 i.v. bolus on day 1 every 3 weeks [51]. In a total of 200 patients, response rates were 27%, 19%, and 11%, respectively. The difference between the first and the latter regimens was significant ($p = 0.03$) in terms of response but not in terms of survival. This study strongly suggests that CTX and VCR do not add activity to DX, while replacing DX DACT with DX results in significantly decreased activity in such a way that one might expect VCR, CTX, and DACT to have very limited value in the treatment of soft tissue sarcomas.

The GOG [52] randomly compared DX 60 mg/m^2 every 3 weeks, with DX 60 mg/m^2 plus CTX 500 mg/m^2 every 3 weeks in a total of 104 patients with uterine sarcomas. Both regimens resulted in a 19% response rate, again indicating that CTX does not add to DX.

The data above suggest that combination chemotherapy only results in improved response rates in comparison with single-agent DX if DX is combined with DTIC.

The ADIC regimen was tested against the same regimen plus either CTX or DACT in a SWOG study [53]. Patients were randomized to receive DX 60 mg/m^2 on day 1 plus DTIC 250 mg/m^2/day on days 1–5 every 3 weeks (the ADIC regimen), or ADIC plus CTX 500 mg/m^2 on day 1 every 3 weeks, or ADIC plus DACT 1.2 mg/m^2 on day 1 every 3 weeks. A total of 276 patients were evaluated. There was no statistically significant difference in response rates of 33%, 34%, and 24%, respectively. Also, median durations of response and survival were not significantly different. Toxicities from each of the treatment arms were equivalent. These data confirm the earlier mentioned ECOG study indicating the very limited value of CTX and DACT in the treatment of adult soft tissue sarcomas.

In an effort to lessen toxicity of the ADIC regimen, the SWOG initiated a study using a different schedule of DTIC administration [54]. The regimen consisted of DX 60 mg/m^2 i.v. on day 1 and DTIC 750 mg/m^2 as a 45-min infusion on day 1. Courses were administered at 21-day intervals. With 10 complete and 17 partial remissions in 114 evaluable patients, the overall response rate was 24%. Indeed, this regimen appeared to be very well tolerated with only moderate myelosuppression and moderate nausea and vomiting.

Recently, the SWOG presented the preliminary data from a randomized trial comparing the effectiveness of bolus versus continuous infusion administration of DX and DTIC [55]. The toxicity appeared to be reduced by the infusion regimen (104 evaluable patients) as compared with the bolus regimen (112 evaluable patients), while response rates were 22% and 23%, respectively.

Since 1972, the SWOG has reported several studies including the original ADIC regimen. A remarkable observation is the constant decrease in response rate over the years, starting with 42% and now at 23%. This might be related to the improvement in diagnostic techniques enabling a better evaluation of true responses.

Although the earlier discussed ECOG, GOG, and SWOG studies on combination chemotherapy regimens [51–53] and the single-agent data generated by the EORTC [29] at the moment do not support the inclusion of CTX in combination chemotherapy regimens, this drug together with VCR was incorporated with ADIC, resulting in the CYVADIC regimen [cyclophosphamide (Cytoxan)–vincristine–Adriamycin (doxorubicin)–DTIC] originally studied in M.D. Anderson Hospital and afterward adapted by several other groups.

The original CYVADIC regimen consisted of CTX 500 mg/m^2 i.v. on day 1, VCR 1.5 mg/m^2 i.v. on days 1 and 5, DX 50 mg/m^2 i.v. on day 1, and DTIC 250 mg/m^2/day i.v. on days 1–5 [56]. In the initial 125 patients studied, 21 complete remissions (CRs) (17%) and 42 partial remissions (PRs) (34%) were achieved. The median duration was 9½ months for CR and 7 months for PR. In subsequent follow-up reports including more patients, the response rate did not change [57, 58]. One of the important observations within this study was that the CR rate was much higher in patients <50 years of age than in those >50 [57]. Also, after having treated 331 patients with CYVADIC, the investigators could stress the importance of achieving CR because 21% of those patients had remained disease free for more than 5 years and have been potentially cured by chemotherapy [58]. Finally, also patients in PR who could be converted to CR experienced long-term survival, suggesting cure [58].

The only randomized study including CYVADIC that has been completed was reported by Pinedo et al. [59] on behalf of the EORTC group. It compared CYVADIC (CTX 500 mg/m^2 i.v. on day 1, VCR 1.5 mg/m^2 on day 1, and DX 50 mg/m^2/day on days 1–5 every 4 weeks with a schedule alternating VCR/ CTX and ADIC in similar doses as used with CYVADIC, at 4-week intervals. With CYVADIC, 17% CRs and 21% PRs were achieved in 84 patients while, in the cycling arm, a significantly lower response rate of 5% CR and 9% PR was achieved in 78 patients ($p = 0.001$), reflecting the lower activity of CTX/ VCR as compared with ADIC, which suggests that patients with soft tissue sarcomas do not benefit from alternating non-cross-resistant combinations of the currently known drugs, confirming results of earlier trials [60, 61]. More-over, the EORTC results indicate that DX should be administered every 3 or 4 weeks instead of every 8 weeks [59].

Other studies have confirmed the activity of CYVADIC [62–64]. The regimen induces nausea and/or vomiting in almost all patients, as well as alopecia. Also leukocytopenia and thrombocytopenia appear to be substantial, but the regimen nevertheless is considered tolerable. The disadvantage of both the original ADIC and CYVADIC regimens is the necessity of hospitalization. To reduce the required number of treatment days and in an effort to reduce toxicity, shorter schedules have been studied [54, 64] (EORTC study 62851). Response rates and toxicity of these shortened treatments appear comparable to those of the original regimens (Table 5), but proof from a randomized trial is not available.

After confirmation of the activity of IFOS in soft tissue sarcomas [29], this drug was combined with DX. The Royal Marsden Group has treated 50 patients with DX 40–60 mg/m^2 i.v. on day 1 plus IFOS 5–8 g/m^2 by 24-h infusion on day 1 with mesna uroprotection [28], with courses repeated every 3 weeks. In 57 evaluable patients, they achieved 6 CRs (11%) and 11 PRs (19%) for an overall response rate of 30%. The optimal doses for the combination appeared to be DX 50 mg/m^2 and IFOS 5 g/m^2. Using that schedule, the EORTC Soft Tissue and Bone Sarcoma Group performed a phase II trial [65]. In 178 evaluable patients, 16 CRs (9%) and 47 PRs (26%) were noted

Table 5. Various schedules of DTIC infusion in ADIC and CYVADIC combination chemotherapy

Regimen	DTIC (days of treatment)	Total DTIC dose (mg/m^2)	No. of evaluable patients	Response rate (%)			Ref.
				CR	PR	Overall	
ADIC	1–5	1250	237	11	24	35	8, 23, 26, 27
	1	750	114	9	15	24	27
CYVADIC	1–5	1250	314	16	26	42	30, 32, 35, 36
	1–3	1200	60	7	42	49	37

Table 6. Combination chemotherapy: most extensively studied combinations

Drugs	No. of evaluable* patients	Response rate (%)			Ref.
		CR	PR	Overall	
DX–DTIC	351	10	21	31	8, 23, 26, 27
DX–DTIC–CTX–VCR	374	14	29	43	32, 35–37
DX–IFOS	235	9	25	34	38, 39

* Cumulative data.

for an overall response rate of 35%, in fact confirming the Royal Marsden data. The major toxicities were leukopenia, nausea and vomiting, and alopecia, all of which were manageable. Currently, the EORTC group is conducting a randomized trial comparing the DX–IFOS regimen with single-agent DX 75 mg/m^2 i.v. on day 1 every 3 weeks, and with CYVADIC administered 1 day every 3 weeks.

Other combinations have been studied, but none appeared to be superior to ADIC, CYVADIC, or DX–IFOS [66], and it is difficult to conclude which of these three is the best. Therefore, the results of the ongoing EORTC study are awaited with interest. In the meantime, it seems justified to use CYVADIC as standard regimen in patients treated outside of trials because, despite the absence of single-agent CTX and VCR activity, the reported studies indicate the highest overall response rate and, even more important, the highest CR rate with this regimen (Table 6). The CR patients may potentially be cured by chemotherapy [58], so it appears important to aim at achieving CR.

With the conclusion that DX, IFOS, and DTIC are the only active single agents in the treatment of soft tissue sarcomas, it seems logical to combine these three drugs. Indeed, at Dana Farber Cancer Institute, the first results of the use of such a combination are now available. A phase I study indicated that the maximum tolerated dose was DX 60 mg/m^2, DTIC 900 mg/m^2, and IFOS 7500 mg/m^2 per course when all were given together as a 72-h continuous infusion every 3 weeks [67]. Dose-limiting toxicity was leukopenia.

With antiemetics, Grade-3 nausea and vomiting were infrequent. Other toxicities were remarkably mild. Using this regimen in a phase II study of 62 evaluable patients [68], 6 CRs (10%) and 26 PRs (42%) were achieved. Several other study groups have recently started phase II studies with modified schedules of this three-drug combination.

Prognostic factors

With several study reports available that deal with the three major combination chemotherapy regimens that appear to be comparable as far as response rates are concerned, it becomes possible to obtain further insight into factors predicting the outcome of chemotherapy.

Although several authors indicate that some tumor types may be more responsive than others, Table 7, combining all data of studies with ADIC-based regimens, indicates the opposite. There is no evidence of one histological subtype with a better prognosis.

Regarding other factors with a possible influence on achievement of response there is certainly no consensus on age, sex, and bone marrow reserve. The most important prognostic factor for response appears to be the performance score [8, 57, 59, 64], which may be partly related to a favorable influence of a <5% weight loss [8, 30]. Another important observation from virtually all studies concerns the time necessary to achieve response. The median time varies from 7 to 10 weeks [8, 50, 56, 59, 65], but it is even more important to realize that treatment periods as long as 32 [56], 56 [8], or 101 [59] weeks may be required to achieve response, indicating that soft tissue sarcomas respond rather slowly to chemotherapy.

Mixed mesodermal sarcomas

As has been indicated, cisplatin (CDDP, or *cis*-diamminedichloroplatin) can be considered an inactive single agent for the treatment of soft tissue sarcomas, which has been confirmed by the absence of an additive effect of CDDP when combined with active drugs [63, 69–71]. In contrast to these general data, mixed mesodermal sarcomas (MMS) appear to respond to some extent to CDDP. In a phase II trial with single-agent CDDP at a dose of 50 mg/m² every 3 weeks as second-line chemotherapy, five (18%) of 28 patients achieved a response [45] and, at a higher dose, Gershenson et al. even achieved a 28% response rate [46] (Table 4). These data in MMS appear to be confirmed by limited data on combination chemotherapy including CDDP. Piver et al. [72] combined DTIC and different dosages of CDDP, achieving three responses (27%) in 11 patients. Although DX appears to be less active in MMS than in other histological subtypes [47, 50], others have combined DX and CDDP. Seltzer et al. [73] applied 50 mg/m² DX plus 50 mg/m² CDDP both i.v. on

Table 7. Response rates in histological subtypes of soft tissue sarcomas

Histology	Regimen								
	ADIC			CYVADIC					Total
	[8][a]	[26]	[27]	[29]	[32]	[35]	[37]		
	n^b (%)^c	n (%)	n (%)	n (%)	n (%)	n (%)	n (%)		n (%)
Leiomyosarcoma	27 (44)	73 (33)	27 (19)	31 (58)	35 (20)	18 (22)	6 (17)		217 (33)
MFH	24 (25)	43 (21)	13 (54)	—	29 (34)	5 (40)	6 (67)		120 (32)
Schwannoma	9 (22)	—	—	—	—	—	2 (50)		11 (27)
Liposarcoma	7 (14)	16 (19)	—	12 (41)	15 (33)	5 (40)	4 (25)		59 (29)
Fibrosarcoma	4 (0)	—	6 (50)	21 (48)	19 (37)	2 (50)	9 (56)		61 (43)
Synoviasarcoma	3 (0)	10 (33)	2 (0)	2 (50)	7 (28)	—	9 (67)		30 (33)
Angiosarcoma	—	12 (25)	—	5 (60)	7 (14)	—	—		26 (26)
Neurosarcoma	—	12 (33)	10 (20)	13 (69)	6 (17)	—	—		41 (39)
Rhabdomyosarcoma	—	14 (29)	8 (25)	13 (54)	4 (25)	5 (40)	9 (44)		53 (38)

[a] [ ], reference.
[b] n, number of evaluable patients.
[c] (%), response rate.

day 1 every 3 weeks, achieving 3 CRs and 2 PRs in six patients. The Toronto group [74] treated 15 patients with MMS of the ovary with either CAP [CTX, Adriamycin (DX), and Platinol (CDDP)] or CYVADIC achieving a 60% response rate. Jansen et al. [75] achieved five remissions in six patients, with a combination of cyclophosphamide, hexamethylmelamine, doxorubicin, and cisplatin (CHAP-5). Of course, for the latter two studies, we should also consider the possible role of CTX, because this drug may also be active in MMS [29]. In the near future, the role of CDDP as well as CTX in this rare, but less-DX-responsive, sarcoma subtype should be explored.

Induction chemotherapy

The value of preoperative chemotherapy in the treatment of locally far-advanced soft tissue sarcomas is one of the important issues of investigation in the present decade. Intra-arterial chemotherapy is discussed in Chapter 8 by Huth and Eilber. As for other tumor types, there is also increasing interest in systemic induction chemotherapy for which only limited data are yet available, usually as case reports. However, Rouëssé et al. [76] recently reported a series of 34 patients with locally far-advanced, but nonmetastatic, sarcomas treated with either DX–CTX–CDDP–DTIC–vindesine (DCPAV), CYVADIC, or DX–IFOS, achieving 38% remissions: 24 patients underwent surgery after 2–7 cycles of chemotherapy, which in 12 proved to be radical. Patients who did not undergo radical operation were irradiated postoperatively. While 2-year survival was only 18% in those patients who never achieved CR, it was 80% in patients who achieved CR after chemotherapy + surgery + radiotherapy, a figure at least suggesting a benefit of preoperative systemic chemotherapy (Fig. 1). Also, at Dana Farber Cancer Institute, some patients were

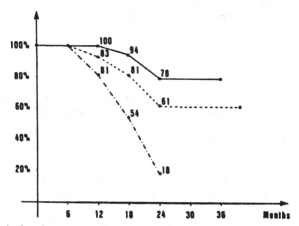

Figure 1. Survival of patients responding to systemic preoperative chemotherapy versus those not responding: (—) patients with CR, *n* = 22; (----) total number of patients, *n* = 34; and (—·—·) patients without a CR, *n* = 12. Reproduced from Rouëssé et al. [76], with permission.

treated with DX–IFOS–DTIC preoperatively [68]. During the 1987 ASCO meetings, there were preliminary reports of an 82% response rate in a limited number of patients. Clearly this type of treatment should be further explored.

Conclusion

The last few years have shown a trend toward consensus in the chemotherapeutic approach of soft tissue sarcomas. Three active single agents—DX, IFOS, and DTIC—are available. CTX and CDDP may also be considered active in the treatment of mixed mesodermal sarcomas. The ECOG study comparing DX with ADIC indicates that combination chemotherapy yields higher response rates than does single-agent chemotherapy, although other studies applying inactive combination regimens previously suggested the opposite. Therefore the results of the ongoing randomized EORTC study are awaited with interest. At this moment, there is no proof that combination chemotherapy also yields improved survival when compared with single-agent treatment.

Although it is not clear which combination chemotherapy is the best, three regimens emerge as most interesting: ADIC, CYVADIC, and DX–IFOS. Although the addition of CTX and VCR to ADIC still can be debated, non-randomized studies suggest that CYVADIC yields the highest CR rate, which may be important because of indications that these patients may potentially be cured. The future years will highlight investigations on the combination DX–IFOS–DTIC.

The role of systemic preoperative chemotherapy will also have to be further outlined, because preliminary data indicate high response rates. However, regarding this topic, survival will be more important than response.

Clearly there is still a need for new active drugs and therefore the continuous search through phase II trials should be encouraged.

References

1. Enneking WF, Spanier SS, Malawer MM: The effect of the anatomic setting on the results of surgical procedures for soft-part sarcomas of the thigh. Cancer 47:1005–1022, 1981.
2. Lindberg RD, Martin RG, Ramsdahl MM: Surgery and postoperative radiotherapy in the treatment of soft tissue sarcomas in adults. AJR Ther Nucl Med 123:123–129, 1975.
3. Gerson R, Shiu MH, Hajdu SI: Sarcoma of the buttock: a trend toward limb-salvage resection. J Surg Oncol 19:238–242, 1982.
4. Leibel SA, Tranbaugh RF, Wara WM, et al.: Soft tissue sarcomas of the extremities: survival and patterns of failure with conservative surgery and postoperative irradiation compared to surgery alone. Cancer 50:1076–1083, 1982.
5. Suit HD, Mankin HJ, Wood WC, Proppe KH: Preoperative, intraoperative, and postoperative radiation in the treatment of primary soft tissue sarcoma. Cancer 55:2659–2667, 1985.
6. Bonadonna G, Beretta G, Tancini G, et al.: Adriamycin (NSC-123127) studies at the Instituto Nazionale Tumori, Milan. Cancer Chemother Rep 6:231–245, 1975.

7. Verweij J, van Oosterom AT, Pinedo HM: Melanomas, soft tissue and bone sarcomas. Eur J Cancer Clin Oncol [Suppl] 4:75–85, 1985.
8. Borden EC, Amato DA, Rosenbaum Ch, et al.: Randomized comparison of three adriamycin regimens for metastatic soft tissue sarcomas. J Clin Oncol 5:840–850, 1987.
9. O'Bryan RM, Luce JK, Talley RW: Phase II evaluation of adriamycin in human neoplasma. Cancer 32:1–8, 1973.
10. Mitts DL, Gerhardt H, Armstrong D, et al.: Chemotherapy for advanced soft tissue sarcomas: results of phase I and II cooperative studies. Tex Med 75:43–47, 1979.
11. Chlebowski RT, Paroly WS, Pugh RP: Adriamycin given as a weekly schedule without a loading course: clinically effective with reduced incidence of cardiotoxicity. Cancer Treat Rep 64:49–51, 1980.
12. Gerlach JH, Bell DR, Karakousis C, et al.: P-glycoprotein in human sarcoma: evidence for multidrug resistance. J Clin Oncol 5:1452–1460, 1987.
13. Benjamin RS, Yap BS: Infusion chemotherapy for soft tissue sarcomas. In: Baker LH (ed), Soft tissue sarcomas. Boston: Martinus Nijhoff, 1983, pp 109–116.
14. Bramwell VHC, Mouridsen HT, Mulder JH, Somers R, van Oosterom AT, Santoro A, Thomas D, Sylvester R, Markham D: Carminomycin vs adriamycin in advanced soft tissue sarcomas: an EORTC randomized phase II study. Eur J Cancer Clin Oncol 19:1097–1104, 1983.
15. Mouridsen HT, Bastholt L, Somers R, Santoro A, Bramwell V, Mulder JH, van Oosterom AT, Buesa J, Pinedo HM, Thomas D, Sylvester R: Adriamycin versus epirubicin in advanced soft tissue sarcomas: a randomized phase II/phase III study of the EORTC Soft Tissue and Bone Sarcoma Group. Eur J Cancer Clin Oncol 23:1477–1483, 1987.
16. Bodey GP, Yap BS, Ajani J: Clinical trials of 4'-epidoxorubicin. In: Proceedings of the 13th international congress on chemotherapy 215:23–26, 1983.
17. Bertrand M, Multhauf P, Bartolucci A, Ellison D, Gockerman J: Phase II study of acla-rubicin in previously untreated patients with advanced soft tissue sarcoma: a South-Eastern Cancer Study Group trial. Cancer Treat Rep 69:725–726, 1985.
18. Raymond V, Magill GB, Wissel PS, Cheng EW, Ochoa M, Young CW: Phase II trial of deoxydoxorubicin in patients with soft tissue sarcoma. Proc Am Soc Clin Oncol 5:146, 1986.
19. Wissel PS, Magill GB, Raymond V, Well S, Sordillo P, Cheng E: 4'Demethoxydaunorubicin in advanced soft tissue sarcomas: an update with emphasis on patients without prior doxo-rubicin. Proc Am Soc Clin Oncol 3:259, 1984.
20. Presant CA, Gans R, Bartolucci AA: Treatment of metastatic sarcomas with mitoxantrone. Cancer Treat Rep 68:813–814, 1984.
21. Bull FE, von Hoff DD, Balcerzak SP, Stephens RL, Panetierre FJ: Phase II trial of mitoxan-trone in advanced sarcomas: a South-West Oncology Group study. Cancer Treat Rep 69:231–233, 1985.
22. Gottlieb JA, Benjamin RS, Baker LH, et al.: Role of DTIC (NSC-45338) in the chemo-therapy of sarcomas. Cancer Treat Rep 60:199–203, 1976.
23. Buesa J, Mouridsen H, van Oosterom AT, Steward WT, Verweij J, Thomas D: High-dose DTIC in advanced soft tissue sarcoma of the adult: a phase II study of the EORTC Soft Tissue and Bone Sarcoma Group. Proc ECCO 4:235, 1987.
24. Hoefer-Janker H, Scheef W, Gunther U, et al.: Erfahrungen mit der fraktionierten Ifosfamid-Stoss Therapie bei generalisierten malignen Tumoren. Med Welt 26:972–979, 1977.
25. Klein HO, Wickramanayake PD, Coerper CL, et al.: High-dose ifosfamide and mesna as continuous infusion over five days: a phase I/II trial. Cancer Treat Rev 10:167–173, 1983.
26. Czownicki A, Utracka-Hutka B: Contribution to the treatment of malignant tumours with ifosfamide. In: Burkert H, Voight HC (eds), Proceedings of the international Holoxan sym-posium. Düsseldorf: ASTA-Werke, 1977, pp 109–111.
27. Antman KM, Montella D, Rosenbaum Ch, Schwen M: Phase II trial of ifosfamide with mesna in previously treated metastatic sarcoma. Cancer Treat Rep 69:499–504, 1985.
28. Wiltshaw E, Westbury G, Harmer C, McKinna A, Fisher C: Ifosfamide plus mesna with and without adriamycin in soft tissue sarcoma. Cancer Chemother Pharmacol [Suppl 2] 18:

90

S10-12, 1986.

29. Bramwell VHC, Mouridsen H, Santoro A, Blackledge G, Somers R, Verweij J, Dombernowsky P, Onsrud M, Thomas D, Sylvester R, van Oosterom AT: Cyclophosphamide versus ifosfamide: final report of a randomized phase II trial in adult soft tissue sarcomas. Eur J Cancer Clin Oncol 23:311-321, 1987.

30. Sordillo PP, Magill GB, Welt S: Phase II trial of methylglyoxal-bis-guanylhydrazone (methyl-GAG) in patients with soft-tissue sarcomas. Am J Clin Oncol (CCT) 8:316-318, 1985.

31. Thigpen JT, Blessing JA, Homesley HD, Hacker N, Curry SL: Phase II trial of piperazine-dione in patients with advanced or recurrent uterine sarcoma: a Gynecologic Oncology Group Study. Am J Clin Oncol (CCT) 8:350-352, 1985.

32. Amato DA, Borden EC, Shiraki M, Enterline HT, Rosenbaum C, Davis HL, Paul AR, Stevens CM, Lerner HJ: Evaluation of bleomycin, chlorozotocin, MGBG, and bruceantin in patients with advanced soft tissue sarcoma, bone sarcoma, and mesothelioma. Invest New Drugs 3:397-401, 1985.

33. Chan C, Bartolucci A, Brenner D, Presant C, Davila E, Carpenter J, Greco A, Clamon G, Moore J: Phase II trial of diaziquone in anthracycline-resistant adult soft tissue and bone sarcoma patients: a South-Eastern Cancer Study Group trial. Cancer Treat Rep 70:427-428, 1986.

34. Cowan JD, Gehan E, Rivkin SE, Jones SE: Phase II trial of bisantrene in patients with advanced sarcoma: a South-West Oncology Group study. Cancer Treat Rep 70:685-686, 1986.

35. Wissel P, Magill G, Sordillo P, Cheng E, Hakes T, Applewhite A: A phase II trial of mitomycin C in advanced soft tissue sarcomas. Proc Am Soc Clin Oncol 5:146, 1986.

36. Ajani JA, Dimery I, Chawla SP, Pinnamaneni K, Benjamin RS, Legha S, Krakoff IH: Phase II studies of homoharringtonine in patients with advanced malignant melanomas, sarcoma, and head and neck, breast and colorectal carcinomas. Cancer Treat Rep 70:375-379, 1986.

37. Thigpen JT, Blessing JA, Wilbanks GD: Cisplatin as second-line chemotherapy in the treatment of advanced or recurrent leiomyosarcoma of the uterus: a phase II trial of the Gynecologic Oncology Group. Am J Clin Oncol (CCT) 9:18-20, 1986.

38. Sordillo PP, Magill GB, Brenner J, Cheng EW, Dosik M, Yagoda A: A phase II evaluation of cisplatin in previously untreated patients with soft tissue sarcomas. Cancer 59:884-886, 1987.

39. Budd GT, Balcerzak S, Mortimer J, Fletcher W: SWOG 8465: high-dose cisplatin for advanced sarcomas. Proc Am Soc Clin Oncol 6:137, 1987.

40. Rouëssé JG, van Oosterom AT, Capellaere P, Kerbrat P, van Groeningen CJ, Thomas D, Benshahar D: Phase II study of 1,2,4-triglycidyl urasol (TGU) in advanced soft tissue sarcoma: a trial of the EORTC Soft Tissue and Bone Sarcoma Cooperative Group. Eur J Cancer Clin Oncol 23:1413-1414, 1987.

41. Dombernowsky P, Buesa J, Pinedo HM, Santoro A, Mouridsen HT, Somers R, Bramwell V, Onsrud M, Rouëssé J, Thomas D, Sylvester R: VP-16 in advanced soft tissue sarcoma: a phase II study of the EORTC Soft Tissue and Bone Sarcoma Group. Eur J Cancer Clin Oncol 23:579-580, 1987.

42. Zalupski M, Pazdur R, Samson M, Baker L: Phase II clinical evaluation of fludarabine in soft tissue and osteosarcomas. Proc Am Soc Clin Oncol 6:135, 1987.

43. Harris J, Das Gupta T, Vogelzang N, Badrinath K, Bonomi P, Desser R, Locker G, Blough R, Johnson C: Treatment of soft tissue sarcoma with fibroblast interferon (beta-interferon): an American Cancer Society/Illinois Cancer Council study. Cancer Treat Rep 70:293-294, 1986.

44. Edmonson JH, Long HJ, Creagan ET, Frytak S, Sherwin SA, Chang MN: Phase II study of recombinant gamma-interferon in patients with advanced non-osseous sarcomas. Cancer Treat Rep 71:211-213, 1987.

45. Thigpen JT, Blessing JA, Orr JW, DiSaia J: Phase II trial of cisplatin in the treatment of patients with advanced or recurrent mixed mesodermal sarcomas of the uterus: a Gynecologic Oncology Group study. Cancer Treat Rep 70:271-274, 1986.

46. Gershenson DM, Kavanagh JJ, Copeland LJ, Edwardo CL, Stringer CA, Wharton JT: Cisplatin therapy for disseminated mixed mesodermal sarcoma of the uterus. J Clin Oncol 5:618–621, 1987.

47. Morrow CP, Bundy BN, Hoffman J, Sutton G, Homesley H: Adriamycin chemotherapy for malignant mixed mesodermal tumor of the ovary: a Gynecologic Oncology Group study. Am J Clin Oncol (CCT) 9:24–26, 1986.

48. Slayton E, Blessing JA, DiSaia PJ, Christopherson WA: Phase II trial of etoposide in the management of advanced or recurrent mixed mesodermal sarcomas of the uterus: a Gynecologic Oncology Group study. Cancer Treat Rep 71:661–662, 1987.

49. Gottlieb JA, Baker LH, Quagliana JM, Luce JK, Whitecar JP, Sinkovics JG, Rivkin SE, Brownlee R, Frei E: Chemotherapy of sarcomas with a combination of adriamycin and dimethyl triazeno imidazole carboxamide. Cancer 30:1632–1638, 1972.

50. Omura GA, Major FJ, Blessing JA, Sedlacek TV, Thigpen JT, Creasman WT, Zaino RJ: A randomized study of adriamycin with and without dimethyl triazenoimidazole carboxamide in advanced uterine sarcomas. Cancer 52:626–632, 1983.

51. Schoenfeld DA, Rosenbaum Ch, Horton J, Wolter JM, Falkson G, De Conti RC: A comparison of adriamycin versus vincristine and adriamycin and cyclophosphamide versus vincristine, actinomycin-D and cyclophosphamide for advanced sarcoma. Cancer 50:2757–2762, 1982.

52. Muss HB, Bundy B, DiSaia PJ, Homesley HD, Fowler WC, Creasman W, Yordan E: Treatment of recurrent or advanced uterine sarcoma: a randomized trial of doxorubicin versus doxorubicin and cyclophosphamide (a phase III trial of the Gynecologic Oncology Group). Cancer 55:1648–1653, 1985.

53. Baker LH, Frank J, Fine G, Balcerak SP, Stephens RL, Stuckey WJ, Rivkin S, Saiki J, Ward JH: Combination chemotherapy using adriamycin, DTIC, cyclophosphamide and actinomycin-D for advanced soft tissue sarcomas: a randomized comparative trial—a phase III Southwest Oncology Group study (7613). J Clin Oncol 5:851–861, 1987.

54. Saiki JH, Baker LH, Rivkin SE, Shahbender S, Fletcher WS, Athens JW, Balcerak SP, Bonnet JD: A useful high-dose intermittent schedule of adriamycin and DTIC in the treatment of advanced sarcomas. Cancer 58:2196–2197, 1986.

55. Baker LH, Green S, Ryan J, Rosenberg B, Balcerak S: SWOG 8024: combind modality therapy for disseminated soft tissue sarcoma, phase III. Proc Am Soc Clin Oncol 6:138, 1987.

56. Yap BS, Baker LH, Sinkovics JG, Rivkin SE, Bottomley R, Thigpen T, Burgess MA, Benjamin RS, Bodey GP: Cyclophosphamide, vincristine, adriamycin and DTIC (CYVADIC) combination chemotherapy for the treatment of advanced sarcomas. Cancer Treat Rep 64:93–98, 1980.

57. Yap BS, Burgess MA, Sinkovics JG, Benjamin RS, Bodey GP: A 5-year experience with cyclophosphamide, vincristine, adriamycin and DTIC (CYVADIC) chemotherapy in 169 adults with advanced soft tissue sarcoma. Proc Am Soc Clin Oncol 22:534, 1981.

58. Yap BS, Sinkovics JG, Burgess MA, Benjamin RS, Bodey GP: The curability of advanced soft tissue sarcomas in adults with chemotherapy. Proc Am Soc Clin Oncol 2:239, 1983.

59. Pinedo HM, Bramwell VHC, Mouridsen H, Somers R, Vendrik CPJ, Santoro A, Buesa J, Wagener Th, van Oosterom AT, van Unnik JAM, Sylvester R, de Pauw M, Thomas D, Bonadonna G: CYVADIC in advanced soft tissue sarcoma: a randomized study comparing two schedules. Cancer 53:1825–1832, 1984.

60. Dalley DN, Levi JA, Nesbitt RA, Tattersall MHM, Woods RL, Fox RM, Aroney RS: Cyclical combination chemotherapeutic regimen in adult soft tissue sarcoma. Cancer Clin Trials 4:163–165, 1981.

61. Presant CA, Lowenbraun S, Bartolucci AA, Smalley RV, the Southeastern Cancer Study Group: Metastatic sarcoma: chemotherapy with adriamycin, cyclophosphamide and methotrexate alternating with actinomycin-D, DTIC and vincristine. Cancer 47:457–465, 1981.

62. Karakousis CP, Rao U, Park HG: Combination chemotherapy (CYVADIC) in metastatic soft tissue sarcomas. Eur J Cancer Clin Oncol 18:33–36, 1982.

63. Kerzel W, König HJ, Walter M, Arnold I: Zytostatische Kombinationsbehandlung fort-

geschrittener Sarkome: Ergebnisse einer prospektiv angelegten Studie. Tumor Diagn Ther 6:180–184, 1985.

64. Bui NB, Chauvergne J, Hocke C, Durand M, Brunet R, Coindre JM: Analysis of a series of sixty soft tissue sarcomas in adults treated with a cyclophosphamide–vincristine–adriamycin–dacarbazine (CYVADIC) combination. Cancer Chemother Pharmacol 15:82–85, 1985.

65. Schuette J, Mouridsen H, Santoro A, Steward W, van Oosterom AT, Somers R, Blackledge G, Verweij J, Rouëssé J, Green JA, Pinedo HM, Kaye SB, Kerbrat H, Wagener T, Thomas D, Sylvester R: Adriamycin and ifosfamide, a new effective combination in advanced soft tissue sarcoma. Proc ECCO 4:232, 1987.

66. Pinedo HM, Verweij J: The treatment of soft tissue sarcomas with focus on chemotherapy: a review. Radiother Oncol 5:193–205, 1986.

67. Elias AD, Antman KH: Doxorubicin, ifosfamide and dacarbazine (AID) with mesna uroprotection for advanced untreated sarcoma: a phase I study. Cancer Treat Rep 70:827–833, 1986.

68. Elias AD, Ryan L, Aisner J, Antman KH: Doxorubicin, ifosfamide and DTIC (AID) for advanced untreated sarcomas. Proc Am Soc Clin Oncol 6:134, 1987.

69. Klippstein TH, Mitrou PS, Kochendörfer KJ, Bergmann L: High-dose adriamycin and cis-platinum in advanced soft tissue sarcomas and invasive thymomas: a pilot study. Cancer Chemother Pharmacol 13:78–81, 1984.

70. Hartlapp JH, Münch HJ, Illinger HJ, Wolter H, Jensen JC: Alternatives to CYVADIC combination therapy of soft tissue sarcomas. Cancer Chemother Pharmacol [Suppl 2] 18: S20–S23, 1986.

71. Edmonson JH, Hahn RG, Schutt AJ, Bisel HF, Ingle JN: Cyclophosphamide, doxorubicin and cisplatin combined in the treatment of advanced sarcomas. Med Pediatr Oncol 11:319–321, 1983.

72. Piver MS, Lele SB, Patsner B: Cis-diamminedichloroplatinum plus dimethyl-triazenoimidazole carboxamide as second- and third-line chemotherapy for sarcomas of the female pelvis. Gynecol Oncol 23:371–375, 1983.

73. Seltzer V, Kaplan B, Vogl S, Spitzer M: Doxorubicin and cisplatin in the treatment of advanced mixed mesodermal uterine sarcoma. Cancer Treat Rep 68:1389–1390, 1984.

74. Moore N, Fine S, Sturgeon J: Malignant mixed mesodermal tumors of the ovary: the Princess Margaret Hospital experience. Proc Am Soc Clin Oncol 5:114, 1986.

75. Jansen RLH, van der Burg MEL, Verweij J, Stoter G: Cyclophosphamide, hexamethylmelamine, adriamycin and cisplatin combination chemotherapy in mixed mesodermal sarcoma of the female genital tract. Eur J Cancer Clin Oncol 23:1131–1133, 1987.

76. Rouëssé JG, Friedman S, Sevin DM, Le Chevalier Th, Spielmann ML, Contesso G, Sarrazin DM, Genin JR: Preoperative induction chemotherapy in the treatment of locally advanced soft tissue sarcomas. Cancer 60:296–300, 1987.

7. Adjuvant chemotherapy for soft tissue sarcomas

Vivien H.C. Bramwell

There has been steady progress in the management of soft tissue sarcomas, particularly those located in extremities, which comprise ~60% of the total. The judicious use of multimodality therapy has improved functional outcome without sacrifice of local control.

The role of chemotherapy in controlling systemic micrometastasis remains an extremely controversial issue, and the results of studies published since Volume 2 of this series have not, with one possible exception [1], demonstrated convincingly that adjuvant chemotherapy can reduce the incidence of metastases.

Soft tissue sarcomas are rare tumors, and adjuvant chemotherapy studies that have accrued more than 100 patients are the exception rather than the rule. To enhance uniformity, many studies have concentrated on high-grade extremity sarcomas, but this has further restricted numbers. Although it is generally acknowledged that histological grade is the most important prognostic factor, several very distinct grading systems are in use [2–5], dividing tumors into two, three, or four categories. There is no uniformly accepted staging system, although those proposed by the American Joint Commission for Cancer Staging and End Results Reporting (AJC) [2] and Enneking [6] are most widely used. Thus, comparison of results between studies is very difficult and, for small trials, uniformity between randomized groups, with respect to prognostic factors, cannot be assured.

Randomized trials of adjuvant chemotherapy

As in Volume 2 of this series, this chapter concentrates on a review of randomized studies, particularly those comparing a group receiving adjuvant chemotherapy with a concurrent control group. General criteria of eligibility for these studies have been detailed in Volume 2.

Doxorubicin versus control

Table 1 summarizes the results of five trials [1, 7–10], each of which examines the outcome for a group receiving adjuvant doxorubicin (DX) by compari-

Pinedo, H.M., Verweij, J., eds. TREATMENT OF SOFT TISSUE SARCOMAS.

Table 1. Adjuvant chemotherapy: randomized studies of doxorubicin vs control

Center	Treatment	No. evaluable patients	Median FU months	LR[e]	Mets.[e]	RFS %[e]	OS %[e]
Boston/ECOG[b] [7] (1978–1985)	DX[a]	37	49 (16–80)	3	NS[e]	74 } p = 0.11	68 } p = 0.23
	Control	38		4	NS	62	68
UCLA[c] [8] (1981–1984)	DX	55	30	4	NS	78 } n.s.	NS } n.s.[e]
	Control	59		8	NS	74	NS
Intergroup[b] (USA) [9] (1983–1987)	DX	32	20 (1–39)	NS	NS	67 } n.s.	82 } n.s.
	Control	32		NS	NS	67	89
Scandinavia[b] [10] (1981→)	DX	146	36[d]	NS	NS	NS } p = 0.10	NS
	Control			NS	NS	NS	NS
Bologna[c] [1] (1981→)	DX	33	36[d]	4	7	68 } p < 0.02	88 } p < 0.05
	Control	44		7	22	42	68

[a] DX, doxorubicin.
[b] Sarcomas all sites.
[c] Extremity sarcomas only
[d] Approximate; actual value not stated.
[e] FU, follow-up; LR, local recurrence; Mets., metastases; n.s., not significant; NS, not stated; OS, overall survival; and RFS, relapse-free survival.

son with a randomized control group treated only by surgery with or without radiotherapy.

Boston/ECOG [7]. In 1978, two independent randomized prospective trials of adjuvant DX were initiated by the Dana-Faber Cancer Institute/Massachusetts General Hospital (Boston) and the Eastern Cooperative Oncology Group (ECOG). The detailed protocols were described in Volume 2.

At median follow-up of 49 months (range, 16–80), there were no significant differences between the two arms (Table 1) with respect to local control, metastasis-free survival, relapse-free survival (RFS), and overall survival (OS). Although there was a slight delay in the appearance of metastases in the DX group, the difference was not significant. Subgroup analysis by site showed no evidence of benefit from DX therapy either for extremity (44 patients) or for nonextremity sarcomas. Two patients developed symptomatic DX cardiomyopathy. The authors of this report concluded that "there is no advantage to the use of adjuvant doxorubicin in the treatment of soft tissue sarcoma."

UCLA [8]. This series of protocols from Eilber et al. at the University of California, Los Angeles (UCLA), combining intra-arterial (i.a.) DX and preoperative irradiation, is described in detail in a later section. A cohort of patients in these protocols also entered a prospective randomized study of adjuvant DX (45 mg/m^2/day ×2, q4 weeks, ×5) starting within 6 weeks of surgery. As illustrated in Table 1, at a median follow-up of 30 months, RFS was similar for 55 patients receiving DX and 59 controls. The administration of i.a. DX 60–90 mg by 72-h infusion preoperatively to all patients is a confounding factor, as theoretically this treatment could have had a systemic adjuvant effect, obscuring any difference between the two arms.

Intergroup (USA) [9]. A preliminary report [9] of this study has appeared in abstract form. The DX dose was 70 mg/m^2, q3 weeks, ×6. Of 92 patients randomized, 16 were ineligible and follow-up data were missing on 12, leaving 64 evaluable patients followed for 1–39 months (median, 20), RFS and OS were not significantly different between the two arms, considering extremity and nonextremity subgroups separately, and all eligible patients. Two patients developed symptomatic DX cardiotoxicity.

Scandinavia [10]. The Scandinavian study is the largest study of adjuvant DX, but it also has been reported only in abstract form. Patients with high-grade (Broder's III and IV) sarcomas received DX 60 mg/m^2, q4 weeks, ×9 courses. Over a 4-year period, 156 patients had been accrued, of whom 146 were considered evaluable. Median follow-up was not stated, but would be ~3 years. Data on outcome remained coded and, although RFS was better for one arm of the study, the difference was not significant. OS data were not given.

Bologna [1]. The results of this study, first reported in 1986 [11] and updated at a symposium in 1987 [1], are the only data that support the use of adjuvant DX. There were three surgical groups:

1) *Amputation* (28 patients): Patients were randomized, after immediate ablative surgery, to DX 25 mg/m^2/day ×3 q3 weeks ×6 commencing 3 days postoperatively, or a control group.
2) *Conservative surgery* (29 patients): Biopsy was followed by 45 Gy radiotherapy over 3 weeks combined with two cycles of DX (150 mg/m^2). Definitive surgery was performed and then patients were randomized between chemotherapy—four cycles of DX (300 mg/m^2)—and control groups.
3) *Reexcision* (20 patients): If persistent tumor was suspected, patients treated at another hospital within the previous 3 months had a further excision of the tumor bed, and then were randomized as in group 1. Radiotherapy was given if residual tumor was demonstrated histologically.

The technique of randomization, which used pair-matched stratification for age, site, size of tumor, and stage, led to a large imbalance in patient numbers between DX (24 patients) and control (35 patients) groups at the time of the first report [11], and has been criticized [12]. The study was first reported at 28 months median follow-up, with an accrual of 59 patients, at which time RFS was significantly better for the DX-treated group (79.1% vs 54.3%; $p < 0.005$). Updated figures for 77 patients at ∼3 years of follow-up are shown in Table 1 [1]. Significant differences in RFS ($p < 0.02$) and OS ($p < 0.05$), favoring the DX-treated group, persist.

Comment. Why is there a discrepancy between the results of the Bologna study [1], which to date has accrued 77 patients, and those of four other studies, using similar protocols and collectively registering 399 patients [7–10]? Conventional techniques of statistical analysis accept an alpha error of 5%, which means that, by chance alaone, one in 20 truly negative trials will produce a positive answer, and perhaps this also applies to the Bologna study [1]. Conversely, as acknowledged in the report on the Boston/ECOG study [7], the power to detect a difference in RFS of 20% (60% vs 80%) with a sample size of 75 and follow-up of 49 months is only 57%, and small but important differences may be missed in studies with limited accrual. At present, very limited information is available on the largest trial [10] from Scandinavia, but a full report is awaited with interest.

As outlined in the introduction, tumor grade and size are important prognostic factors used to determine stage. In general, because of anatomical constraints limiting radical surgery, the outcome is worse for nonextremity tumors (with the possible exception of sarcomas of the trunk). All studies shown in Table 1 excluded low-grade sarcomas, although differences in grading classifications make more detailed comparisons between studies difficult. Two studies [1, 8] confined themselves to extremity sarcomas, but, for other studies, extremity tumors were usually analyzed separately. Randomization does not guarantee balance of prognostic factors between compared groups, and the control group of the Bologna study [1] included an excess of pelvis/thigh tumors (57% vs 37.5%), which are generally larger and have a poorer prognosis than distal or upper-extremity tumors. Despite similar durations of follow-up, the RFS (42%) for control patients in the Bologna study is worse than that for comparable control groups of other studies shown in Table 1. Conversely, the RFS (68%) for the DX group is similar to that achieved by chemotherapy and control groups of other studies.

A similar criticism has been leveled against the National Cancer Institute (NCI) randomized trial [13] which has been the only other study to demonstrate significant differences in RFS and OS for patients receiving adjuvant chemotherapy.

Combination chemotherapy versus control

Table 2 summarizes the results of four randomized studies [14–17] evaluating various combination chemotherapies. Details of the chemotherapy dose/schedules have been presented in Volumes 1 and 2 of this series.

M.D. Anderson [14]. This study was performed in the early 1970s and reported by Lindberg et al. [18] in 1976. It was reviewed in Volume 1 of this series. At median follow-up of 18 months, distant metastases had occurred more frequently in the chemotherapy group (9 of 27 vs 3 of 20) and there had been two local recurrences in the control group. RFS did not differ significantly between chemotherapy (67%) and control (85%) groups. Recently, the study has been reanalyzed after 10 years of follow-up [14] and RFS now favors the chemotherapy group, although OS is not significantly different. This discrepancy can be explained by the fact that, although there were fewer local recurrences in the chemotherapy arm, 2 vs 8, metastases occurred with similar frequency in chemotherapy (45%) and control (48%) groups.

Mayo Clinic [15]. This study was discussed in Volume 2 and is summarized in Table 2. As no new data are available, it will not be considered further.

National Cancer Institute [16]. The first randomized study performed by this group has been described in detail in Volumes 1 and 2 and of this series. Updated results [16] are illustrated in Table 2. At a median follow-up of 85 months, for extremity sarcomas, RFS is significantly better, 75% vs 54% ($p = 0.04$), for the chemotherapy group. In contrast with previous reports, the OS figures of 82% and 62% are not significantly different ($p = 0.12$) although they still favor the chemotherapy arm. Local recurrences, 1 vs 4, were less frequent after chemotherapy, but rates of metastases for each group were not specified. A parallel study [19] of nonextremity sarcomas (head, neck, trunk, breast) was discussed in Volume 2, and has not been updated.

Table 2. Adjuvant chemotherapy: randomized studies of combination chemotherapy vs control

Center[b]	Treatment[a]	Site	No. evaluable patients	Median FU months	LR[e]	Mets.[c]	RFS[e] %	OS[e] %
M.D. Anderson [14] (1973–1976)	VCR–DX–CTX–DACT	Limb	20	>120	2	9	54 $p = 0.04$	65 $p = 0.25$
	Control		23		8	11	35	46
Mayo Clinic [15] (1975–1981)	VCR–CTX–DACT alternating VCR–DX–DTIC	Limb / Abdomen[c]	26 / 4	64	17	NS	NS[c] $p = 0.55$	90
	Control	Limb / Abdomen[c]	26 / 5			NS	NS	77
NCI [16] (1977–1981)	DX–CTX–HDMTX	Limb	39	85	1	NS	75 $p = 0.04$	82 $p = 0.12$
	Control		28		4	NS	54	60
	DX–CTX–HDMTX	Head,[d] neck, trunk	17	35	NS	NS	77 $p = 0.08$	68 $p = 0.38$
	Control		14		NS	NS	49	58
EORTC [17] (1978)	CTX–VCR–DX–DTIC	Limb	114	36	9	24	67 $p = 0.06$	77 $p = 0.33$
	Control		119		13	33	57	75
	CTX–VCR–DX–DTIC	Head,[c] neck, trunk	59	36	9	18	61 $p = 0.09$	81 $p = 0.12$
	Control		66		25	17	44	66
	CTX–VCR–DX–DTIC	All	173	36	18	42	67 $p = 0.01$	79 $p = 0.12$
	Control		185		38	50	52	74

a CTX, Cytoxan (cyclophosphamide); DACT, actinomycin D; DTIC, dacarbazine; DX, doxorubicin; CR, vincristine; HDMTX, high dose methotrexate.

b M.D. Anderson, 25% low grade; NCI, no low grade; and EORTC, 18% low grade.

c Includes retroperitoneal.

d Excludes retroperitoneal.

e LR, local recurrence; Mets., metastases; NS, not stated; OS, overall survival; RFS, relapse-free survival; and FU, Follow up.

Building on the results of their previous study, and dismayed by the high incidence of cardiomyopathy, Rosenberg and coworkers went on to compare their "standard" chemotherapy with an abbreviated course of treatment, giving much lower total doses of DX and cyclophosphamide, and omitting high-dose methotrexate [16]. A total of 88 patients entered this trial and, after a median follow-up period of 52 months, 5-year RFS figures were 58% and 72% for high-dose and low-dose chemotherapy arms ($p = 0.37$), respectively, and corresponding figures for OS were 69% and 75% ($p = 0.90$). There were no significant differences in the survival curves for patients receiving high-dose chemotherapy in the two consecutive studies ($p = 0.22$).

EORTC [17]. Preliminary results from this study were published in 1985 [20] and discussed in Volume 2. The study is now in its 10th year of accrual and, with 446 patients on study, is the largest trial of adjuvant chemotherapy in soft tissue sarcomas. The outcome for 358 eligible patients [17] is shown Table 2. Approximately half of the patients received postoperative irradiation and 65% had extremity tumors. Two of the most important prognostic factors—tumor size and grade—were well balanced between the two arms, with 18% of tumors identified as low grade (<3 mitoses/10 high power field (HPF)). Central pathology review demonstrated some imbalance of histological subtypes between the arms, but the significance of this is uncertain, as convincing data linking prognosis to histological subtype independent of grade are lacking in the literature.

Three-year RFS figures are 67% for CYVADIC [cyclophosphosphamide–vincristine (Adriamycin)–DTIC] vs 52% for control ($p = 0.01$). However, OS at 3 years is not significantly different between the two arms: 79% vs 74% ($p = 0.12$). It appears that CYVADIC reduced local recurrence, but did not prevent metastasis ($p = 0.28$). The influence of CYVADIC on local recurrence was most apparent in head, neck, and trunk tumors ($p = 0.038$) rather than limb sarcomas ($p = 0.32$). The incidence of distant metastases was similar in both arms of the study for head, neck, and trunk tumors ($p = 0.97$) and limb sarcomas ($p = 0.20$), and this was paralleled by survival.

Comment. The available results from combination chemotherapy studies are intriguing. Two trials [14, 17] suggest that the most important effect of adjuvant chemotherapy is improved local control rather than reduction of distant metastases. Adjuvant irradiation was not permitted in the Mayo Clinic study [15], which probably accounts for the high overall rates (30%) of local recurrence. In this study, a reduced frequency of metastases was implied by a delay in time to metastasis and fewer operations to remove metastases in the chemotherapy arm, but unfortunately a detailed breakdown of sites of failure was not provided. As discussed in Volume 2, the chemotherapy used was suboptimal. In the NCI study [16] (Table 2), local recurrence was less frequent in the group that received chemotherapy and this was also true for patients receiving DX in the studies from Bologna [1] and UCLA [8], although in each case the numbers involved were small. This trend was not evident in the Boston/ECOG [7] studies, and the relevant data are not available for the Intergroup [9] and Scandinavian studies [10]. The rate of metastasis in the control group was clearly higher in the Bologna study [1], but has not been clearly presented in other reports [7–10, 15, 16]. A detailed comparison of relapse according to site (local vs distant) in future publications would further elucidate the role of adjuvant chemotherapy.

Conclusions

Four studies of adjuvant DX have not demonstrated significant improvements in RFS or OS [7–10], although trends have usually favored the chemotherapy group. The conflicting results of one study [1] may relate to a poor technique of randomization leading to imbalance of prognostic factors in a small study, or may represent a true positive effect missed by other studies, although this seems less likely. Two studies of combination chemotherapy [14, 17] have demonstrated reduced local recurrence, but no difference in the rate of metastases or OS. In the NCI study [16], with longer follow-up, OS is no longer significantly improved by chemotherapy, although RFS remains significantly better. There were fewer local recurrences in the chemotherapy arm, but the comparative rates of metastasis were not clearly stated.

There are many theoretical reasons to support commencing adjuvant chemotherapy as soon as possible after diagnosis and, in reported studies, this time interval was highly variable. It is perhaps significant that chemotherapy was commenced early in the two studies [1, 13] showing the most benefit, although this was also true for the Boston study [7], in which results were negative. In the EORTC trial [17], a median of 6 weeks elapsed between surgery and commencement of chemotherapy. A new EORTC study, in which a group of patients receiving preoperative DX plus ifosfamide (IFOS) is compared with a control group, addresses this issue. The American Intergroup, in a randomized controlled trial, plans to evaluate a dose-intensive combination of DX–IFOS–DTIC (dacarbazine) [21] given to patients after completion of local treatment. Analysis of this study will be complex, as a variety of methods of local control will be permitted in this study, some of which may lead to considerable delay in the initiation of adjuvant chemotherapy.

To summarize, innovative technical advances in the fields of surgery and radiotherapy can now provide high rates of local control and limb salvage for extremity sarcomas, provided patients are treated in major centers that have access to the necessary multidisciplinary expertise. Future research efforts should be concentrated on techniques to eliminate systemic micrometastases, which are responsible for the death of 30%–50% of patients with higher-grade sarcomas.

References

1. Picci P, Bacci G, Gherlinzoni F, Capanna R, Mercuri M, Ruggieri P, Baldini N, Avella M, Pignatti G, Manfrini M: Results on a randomized trial for the treatment of localized soft tissue tumors (STS) of the extremities in adult patients. In: Recent Concepts in Sarcoma Treatment (Proceedings of the Internat Symp on Sarcomas, Tarpon Springs, Florida, 8–10 October 1987). Eds., JR Ryan, LH Baker, Kluwer Academic Pub., Dordrecht, the Netherlands, 1988, pp 144–148.
2. Russell WO, Cohen J, Enzinger F, Hadju SI, Heise H, Martin RG, Meissner W, Miller WT, Schmitz RL, Suit HD: A clinical and pathological staging system for soft tissue sarcomas. Cancer 40:1562–1570, 1977.
3. Costa J, Wesley RA, Glatstein E, Rosenberg SA: The grading of soft tissue sarcomas: results of a clinicohistopathologic correlation in a series of 163 cases. Cancer 53:530–541, 1984.
4. Trojani M, Contesso G, Coindre JM, Rouëssé J, Bui NB, Mascarel A, Goussot JF, David M, Bonichon F, Lagarde C: Soft tissue sarcomas of adults: study of pathological prognostic variables and definition of a histopathological grading system. Int J Cancer 33:37–42, 1984.
5. Enzinger FM, Weiss SW: Soft tissue sarcomas. St Louis: CV Mosby, 1983, pp 1–12.
6. Enneking WF: Staging of musculoskeletal neoplasma. Skeletal Radiol 13:183–194, 1985.
7. Wilson RE, Wood WC, Lerner HL, Antman K, Amato D, Corson JM, Proppe K, Harmon D, Carey R, Greenberger J, Suit H: Doxorubicin chemotherapy in the treatment of soft tissue sarcoma: combined results of two randomized trials. Arch Surg 121:1354–1359, 1986.
8. Eilber FR, Giuliano AE, Huth JF, Morton DL: Adjuvant adriamycin in high grade extremity soft tissue sarcoma: a randomized prospective trial. Proc Am Soc Clin Oncol 5:125, 1986.
9. Antman K, Amato D, Pilepich M, Lerner H, Balcerzak S, Borden E, Baker L: A randomized intergroup trial of adjuvant doxorubicin (DOX) for soft tissue sarcomas (STS): lack of apparent differences between treatment groups. Proc Am Soc Clin Oncol 6:134, 1987.
10. Alvegard TA: Adjuvant chemotherapy with adriamycin in high grade malignant soft tissue sarcoma: a Scandinavian randomized study. Proc Am Soc Clin Oncol 5:125, 1986.
11. Gherlinzoni F, Bacci G, Picci P, Capanna R, Calderoni P, Lorenzi EG, Bernini M, Emiliani E, Barbieri E, Mormand A, Campanacci M: A randomized trial for the treatment of high grade soft tissue sarcomas of the extremities: preliminary observations. J Clin Oncol 4: 552–558, 1986.
12. Sylvester R: Soft tissue sarcomas of the extremities. [lett]. J Clin Oncol 5:321–322, 1987.
13. Rosenberg SA, Chang AE, Glatstein E: Adjuvant chemotherapy for treatment of extremity soft tissue sarcomas: review of the National Cancer Institute experience. Cancer Treat Symp 3:83–88, 1985.
14. Benjamin RS, Terjanian TO, Fenoglio CJ, Barkley HT, Evans HL, Murphy WK, Martin RG: The importance of combination chemotherapy for adjuvant treatment of high risk patients with soft tissue sarcomas of the extremities. In: Adjuvant therapy of cancer V. New York: Grune and Stratton, 1987, pp 735–744.
15. Edmonson JH, Fleming TR, Ivins JC, Burgert EO, Soule EH, O'Connell MJ, Sim FH, Ahmann DL: Randomized study of systemic chemotherapy following complete excision of non-osseous sarcomas. J Clin Oncol 2:1390–1396, 1984.
16. Baker AR, Chang AE, Glatstein E, Rosenberg SA: National Cancer Institute experience in the management of high grade extremity soft tissue Sarcomas. In "Recent Concept in Sarcoma Treatment" Proceeding of the Internat Symp on Sarcomas, Tarpon Springs, Florida, 8–10 October 1987. Eds., JR Ryan, LH Baker, Kluwer Academic Pub., Dordrecht, the Netherlands, 1988, pp 123–130.
17. Bramwell VHC, Rouëssé J, Steward W, Santoro A, Buesa J, Strafford-Koops H, Wagener T, Somers R, Ruka W, Markham D, Burgers M, Van Unnik J, Comtesso G, Thomas D, Sylvester R, Pinedo H: European experience of adjuvant chemotherapy for soft tissue sarcoma: an interim report of a randomized trial of CYVADIC versus control. In: Proceedings

of the international symposium on sarcomas, Tarpon Springs, Florida, 8–10 October 1987. Boston: Martinus Nijhoff, 1988 (in press).

18. Lindberg RD, Murphy WK, Benjamin RS, Sinkovics JG, Martin RG, Romsdhal MM, Jesse RH, Russell HO: Adjuvant chemotherapy in the treatment of primary soft tissue sarcomas: a preliminary report. In: Management of primary bone and soft tissue tumors, Chicago: Year Book Medical, 1976, pp 343–352.

19. Glenn J. Kinsella T, Glatstein E, Tepper J, Baker A, Sugarbaker P, Sindelar W, Roth J, Brennan M, Costa J, Seipp C, Eesley R, Young RC, Rosenberg SA: A randomized prospective trial of adjuvant chemotherapy in adults with soft tissue sarcomas of the head and neck, breast and trunk. Cancer 55:1206–1214, 1985.

20. Bramwell VHC, Rouëssé J, Santoro A, Ruesa J, Somers R, Thomas D, Sylvester R, Pinedo HM: European experience of adjuvant chemotherapy for soft tissue sarcomas: preliminary report of a randomized trial of cyclophosphamide, vincristine, doxorubicin and dacarbazine. Cancer Treat Symp 3:99–108, 1985.

21. Elias AD, Ryan L, Aisner J, Antman K: Doxorubicin, ifosfamide and DTIC (AID) for advanced untreated sarcomas. Proc Am Soc Clin Oncol 6:134, 1987. (ABSTR)

8. Preoperative intra-arterial chemotherapy

James F. Huth and Frederick R. Eilber

Approximately two-thirds of the soft tissue sarcomas arise in the extremities and, following simple excision, they have a propensity for local recurrence that has often resulted in extremity amputation in order to achieve local control. These tumors also tend to develop systemic metastases, primarily to the lung, which is the major cause of mortality.

At the time of initial diagnosis, the vast majority of patients with soft tissue sarcomas have no detectable distant metastases. Therefore, initial therapy is directed at resection of the primary lesion. Methods for the local treatment of soft tissue sarcomas have been modified over the years as we have become aware of the local growth characteristics and histological characteristics of these tumors. These methods are still evolving as we learn more about the usefulness of various forms of therapy as well as their side effects. Recent advances in multimodality treatment of these tumors with preoperative chemotherapy, radiation therapy, and conservative, wide, local excisions have resulted in a decrease of the local recurrence rate to <5% [1].

The local biology of these tumors presents many problems. In addition to the large mass effect, these tumors can extend along fascial planes, often with areas of normal tissue in between islands of tumor cells. The extension poses problems in terms of the extent of radiation therapy or surgical excision required to remove all gross tumor. Although sarcomas do compress vessels or nerves and become intimately associated with bone, they rarely directly invade these structures. The final problem has to do with determining the metastatic potential of various tumors. Sarcomas tend to spread through the bloodstream to the lungs, and rarely metastasize to lymph nodes. An exception to this are the retroperitoneal sarcomas, which have a high potential for metastasizing to the liver. The three factors that are most strongly related to prognosis are (a) grade of the tumor, (b) size of the original lesion, and (c) ability to gain control of the tumor at the local site.

Pinedo, H.M., Verweij, J., eds. TREATMENT OF SOFT TISSUE SARCOMAS.

Historical perspective of prior treatment modalities

Surgery

The early attempts to treat these tumors surgically were almost always followed by local recurrence, because it was not appreciated that the apparent capsule around these tumors was composed of tumor cells and normal tissue that was compressed by the expanding tumor. Since the surgical procedure was enucleation or excision through this pseudocapsule, local recurrence occurred in 90%–95% of patients. Many authors suggested that a wider excision including the pseudocapsule was necessary to avoid local recurrence [2–4]. More extensive operations were devised that included (a) resection of the tumor capsule and (b), because these tumors tended to spread up fascial planes, muscle groups containing the tumor were removed from origin to insertion for a much wider margin of apparently normal tissue (see Chapter 4). Even with these more complete excisions, the local recurrence rate remained high, ~30%–35% [5–10].

Radiation therapy

The results obtained with radiation therapy alone for the treatment of soft tissue sarcomas have been extremely disappointing, with an overall response rate of 20% and a local control rate in the range of 10%–12%. However, patients selected for this type of treatment often had far-advanced disease. To control gross residual disease, the doses had to be very high (6000–8000 cGy), and the complications from subcutaneous fibrosis and neural injury were unacceptable [11, 12].

Suit et al. [13] and Lindberg et al. [14] concluded that radiation therapy would be more efficacious if only microscopic residual disease was left behind. These and subsequent studies showed that patients who received 5000–6000 cGY of radiation therapy *following* a local excision of their tumor had good control in 85% of cases. This improvement in local control eventually resulted in improved overall survival in these patients without the morbidity of an amputation.

Suit et al. [15, 16] treated a series of patients at the Massachusetts General Hospital with 5000–6000 cGy of *preoperative* radiotherapy. Local recurrence rates were low (12%–15%), but there was an increased incidence of postoperative complications in the healing wound. The number of patients who required amputation was greatly reduced to a level of ~2%. Clearly, radiation therapy had a role to play in the treatment of these patients.

Chemotherapy

For many years, there were few, if any, chemotherapeutic agents that were useful in the treatment of soft tissue sarcomas. Cytoxan (cyclophosphamide), vincristine, and actinomycin D were active for alveolar or rhabdomyosarcomas in children [17], but the response rate in adults to this regimen was poor. However, the introduction of doxorubicin changed this picture [18] (see Chapter 6). Although never used as the sole treatment for primary soft tissue sarcomas, doxorubicin has been used in conjunction with other treatment modalities for the treatment of primary tumors, as will be discussed shortly.

Infusion chemotherapy

The discovery of an effective chemotherapeutic agent led investigators to examine the effects of intra-arterial infusion or perfusion into the extremities of patients bearing soft tissue sarcomas. This concept of regional intra-arterial chemotherapy was suggested by Klopp et al. in 1950 [19] after examining local skin toxicity of inadvertant subcutaneous leakage of nitrogen mustard in patients receiving intravenous chemotherapy. The technique of isolation perfusion of an extremity was introduced by Ryan et al. in 1957 [20] and the technique was altered to *hyperthermic* isolated limb perfusion in 1967 by Stehlin et al. [21]. The basic premise of this therapy was to deliver a high concentration of drug into an area that had been excluded from the general circulation by a tourniquet, thus avoiding systemic toxicity especially to the bone marrow. McBride at the M.D. Anderson Hospital [22] and Stehlin [23] reported their results obtained by isolated limb perfusion with LPAM (L-phenylalanine mustard) and actinomycin D in patients with soft tissue sarcomas. The tumor was excised after the drug treatments. They showed that isolated limb perfusion with these relatively inactive drugs was beneficial. The overall local control rate was 80% and the amputation rate was 10%.

These limb perfusion techniques were interesting and had the theoretical advantage of delivering high concentrations of drug to the tumor. However, the technique is limited to patients with extremity tumors in the distal two-thirds of the leg or arm because of the need for application of the tourniquet. The procedure requires use of an operating room and at least 2½ h of a cardiopulmonary pump oxygenator in order to maintain a viable extremity. This, by necessity, limits the duration of exposure of the tumor to the drug to 1–2 h. In addition, doxorubicin (DX), the most active drug against sarcomas, could not be used because of the toxicity to normal tissues when given in high concentrations, and the fact that DX precipitates in the presence of heparin, which is required during extracorporeal bypass.

The concept of presurgical treatment of sarcomas was an attractive one. This allows for the initiation of systemic treatment of the tumor without the delay required for healing of a surgical wound. Effective treatment may allow regression of the primary tumor and facilitate limb salvage. The cells of the periphery of the tumor bed are the best perfused and best oxygenated and would be expected to be the most sensitive to preoperative therapy, and these are the cells that will be in closest proximity to surgical margins after excision.

Pretreatment also allows the clinician an opportunity to evaluate the in vivo sensitivity of the tumor to the chemotherapeutic agent, which may aid in selection of postoperative adjuvant therapy.

Haskell et al. [24] described our first pilot study in which patients with soft tissue sarcoma were treated with continuous intra-arterial DX infusion for 72 consecutive hours prior to excision. A percutaneous intra-arterial catheter was placed by the Seldinger technique into the major arterial supply to the tumor. DX was infused at the rate of 30 mg/day over 24 h for 3 consecutive days. In this original series of ten patients, the technique was shown to be feasible as there were no serious vascular complications. Pathological examination of the resected specimens revealed ~50% necrosis after this therapy. The local control rate was good, but no definitive results could be obtained from this small study. This study did show, however, that DX could be given by continuous infusion in high concentrations with minimal systemic side effects. We learned that the catheter tip needed to be placed in a high-flow vessel in order to avoid the marked skin erythema and muscle necrosis that would occur if the therapy were given in smaller-diameter vessels such as the brachial or popliteal arteries. Injection of flourescein and use of a Woods lamp allowed us to assess the distribution of flow through the arterial line.

Recognizing that radiation was most effective for microscopic disease and that DX was a very effective radiation sensitizer [25], we reasoned that adding radiation immediately after the infusion of DX might enhance the cytotoxic effect of the preoperative therapy. Therefore, the next ten patients were treated with the same regimen of intra-arterial DX, but this treatment was immediately followed by radiation therapy at a dose of 350 cGy/day for 10 days for a total dose of 3500 cGy [26, 27]. The entire extremity was treated to encompass the muscle groups from origin to insertion. A strip of skin was spared opposite the primary tumors. Following completion of therapy, the patients underwent an en bloc resection of their tumor mass without amputation. We found that tumor cell necrosis had increased to 85% following this therapy. There were few intraoperative problems and little radiation fibrosis as a result of this treatment. However, two patients had postoperative wound necrosis from attempts to close the wound primarily under tension.

An additional series of 107 patients was then studied in order to determine the ability of this protocol to prevent local recurrence and salvage a viable extremity [1]. Of 107 patients studied, three (2.5%) had evidence of local recurrence with an overall survival of 65%. All patients in this series had lesions >5 cm in diameter with 60% of lesions >10 cm. All tumors were pathological grade III. Only two patients required amputation because of complications of therapy. However, the postoperative complication rate was ~35% with wound necrosis being the most commonly encountered problem (20%).

In an attempt to reduce the incidence of local would problems, the dose of preoperative radiation therapy was reduced to 1750 cGy in the next 137 patients. With this lower radiation dose, there was less tumor necrosis in the resected specimen, and the local complication rate was reduced to half. However, the incidence of local recurrence increased to 12%. Therefore, the radiation therapy dose was adjusted upward to 2800 cGy in an attempt to improve the local control rate while avoiding the serious complications encountered with the 3500-cGy dose. This has proven to be a satisfactory compromise. The rate of complications has been reduced to 20%, most of which involve minor wound-healing problems that are managed conservatively. Only ten patients required reoperation for complications of the original surgery, and amputation has been required in two patients (2.6%). The overall survival in the combined group of patients is 79% with a follow-up of 1–12 years (median, 3.7 years).

Other investigators have reported the use of intra-arterial infusions using DX and other chemotherapeutic agents. Karakousis et al. at Roswell Park, who studied a series of patients treated by intra-arterial DX administered by slow bolus infusion, reported an average of 33% necrosis using this technique and had no complications of thrombosis [28]. More recently, Karakousis et al. have reported administration of intra-arterial DX into the extremity while blood flow was interrupted by means of a tourniquet [29]. The purpose was to trap the drug in the extremity in order to obtain a more uniform distribution of blood in the tissues of the extremity. A wide excision of the tumor was then carried out, and excellent local control of the tumor was achieved.

Azzarelli et al. reported a series of 13 patients in which DX was given by continuous infusion for 8 days for a total dose of 100 mg/m^2. A resection was performed 6 days following completion of the therapy. Although no *clinical* response was observed (i.e., >50% decrease in size of the tumor mass), nine of 13 tumors showed >50% necrosis in the resected specimen [30]. DiPietro et al. reported a series of 15 patients treated with prolonged intra-arterial infusion of DX. The patients received 0.3 mg/kg/day × 10 days or 0.4 mg/kg every other day for 20 days. They noted clinical responses in 12 of 15 patients with five tumors shrinking to less than half of their original size [31].

Summary

The major factors affecting prognosis of patients with soft tissue sarcomas are local control, size of the primary tumor, and the grade of the tumor. The only factor that can be influenced following appropriate diagnostic procedures is local control. Surgery alone, even radical surgery or amputation, is insufficient to control large, poorly diffentiated tumors in many cases. Preoperative therapy has been shown to be a highly effective method for local disease control.

Intra-arterial therapy appears to have several advantages in the treatment of extremity sarcomas. (1) Intra-arterial therapy results in at least a sixfold increase in the concentration of drug in the blood perfusing the tumor. If combined with proximal occlusion of blood flow (balloon occlusion or tourniquet occlusion), the concentration of drug being delivered to the tumor may increase by 30-fold [32]. This high local concentration of chemotherapy is achieved in most cases without the high systemic toxicity that would be required by intravenous therapy. (2) Chemotherapy infusion prior to surgery allows administration of cytotoxic therapy through an undisturbed blood supply. This allows for an improved effect of therapy at the tumor margin, which is the area at risk for seeding the wound at the time of extirpative surgery. This may facilitate limb salvage in patients with bulky tumors. (3) Responses to this preoperative therapy allows an in vivo evaluation of the efficacy of the drug against the individual tumor. This may aid in determining efficacy of using the drug for postoperative adjuvant therapy. (4) Preoperative therapy allows treatment of the tumor while awaiting construction of custom prostheses, especially in patients with osteosarcomas of the extremities. (5) Even in patients who do not require a prosthesis, preoperative therapy begins systemic treatment without the delay of allowing the patient to recover from major surgery. Since many patients have undetectable metastatic disease at the time of diagnosis, this may eventually result in a longer overall survival for sarcoma patients.

There are some questions about the systemic benefit derived from intra-arterial therapy. Since a significant amount of DX can bind on the first pass through the tumor bed, the dose that reaches the systemic circulation may be insufficient to treat undetectable metastatic disease. We have noted systemic responses in some patients receiving intra-arterial DX who had systemic disease [33]. It appears that other drugs can be given in a high enough dosage intra-arterially that therapeutic levels of drug are found intravenously at the time of infusion. Further studies need to be conducted using concomitant intra-arterial and intravenous combinations of chemotherapy in order to find a combination that can be effective both locally and systemically.

Preoperative therapy enhances local control of extremity soft tissue sarcomas while facilitating limb salvage surgery. Our protocol utilizing intra-arterial DX and radiation therapy has resulted in local disease control in 98% of patients. Many variables need to be considered in further refining this treatment, including intravenous vs intra-arterial therapy, the addition of cisplatin (as is done by Azzarell; et al. [30]) or other agents to the regimen, and further changes in the dosage and scheduling of radiation therapy.

The future should bring some exciting therapeutic changes for patients with soft sarcomas. Improvements in local therapy may enable even more conservative surgical procedures with the achievement of a better functional extremity, better local control of disease, and an improved overall survival.

References

1. Eilber FR, Giuliano AE, Huth JF, Mirra J, Morton DL: Limb salvage for high grade soft tissue sarcomas of the extremity: experience at the University of California, Los Angeles. Cancer Treat Symp 3:49–57, 1985.

2. Bowden L, Booher RJ: The principles and technique of resection of soft parts for sarcoma. Cancer 44:963–977, 1958.

3. Brennhoud IO: The treatment of soft tissue sarcomas: a plea for a more urgent and aggressive approach. Acta Chir Scand 131:438–442, 1966.

4. Pack G: End results in the treatment of sarcomata of the soft somatic tissues. Am J Bone Joint Surg 36:241–263, 1954.

5. Clark RL, Martin RG, White EC: Clinical aspects of soft tissue tumors. Arch Surg 74:859–870, 1957.

6. Gerner RE, Moore GE, Pickren JW: Soft tissue sarcomas. Ann Surg 181:803–808, 1975.

7. Markhede G, Angervoll L, Stenner B: A multivariant analysis of the prognosis after surgical treatment of malignant soft-tissue tumors. Cancer 49:1721–1733, 1981.

8. Martin R, Butler J: Soft tissue tumors: surgical treatment and results. In: Tumors of bone and soft tissue. Chicago: Year Book Medical, 1965, pp 333–347.

9. Rantakokko V, Ekfor TO: Sarcomas of the soft tissue in the extremities and limb girdles. Acta Chir Scand 145:385–394, 1970.

10. Shiu MH, Castro EB, Hajdu SI: Surgical treatment of 297 soft tissue sarcomas of the extremity. Ann Surg 182:597–602, 1975.

11. Windeyer SB, Dische S, Mansfield J: The place of radiation therapy in the management of fibrosarcoma of the soft tissue. Clin Radiol 17:32–40, 1966.

12. McNeer G, Cantin J, Chu F, et al.: Effectiveness of radiation therapy in the management of sarcoma of the somatic soft tissue. Cancer 22:391–397, 1968.

13. Suit HD, Propper KH, Mankin NJ, et al.: Radiation therapy and conservative surgery for sarcoma of soft tissue. Prog Clin Cancer 8:311–318, 1982.

14. Lindberg R, Martin R, Ramsdahl M, et al.: Conservative surgery and postoperative radiotherapy in 300 adults with soft tissue sarcoma. Cancer 47:2391–2397, 1981.

15. Suit HD, Propper KH, Mankin NJ, et al.: Radiation therapy and conservative surgery of sarcoma of soft tissue. Prog Clin Cancer 8:311–318, 1982.

16. Suit HD, Mankin HJ, Wood WC, et al.: Preoperative, intraoperative and postoperative radiation in the treatment of primary soft tissue sarcoma. Cancer 55:2659–2667, 1985.

17. Donaldson S, Castro J, Wilbur J, et al.: Rhabdomysarcoma of the head and neck in children: combination treatment by surgery, irradiation, and chemotherapy. Cancer 31:26–35, 1973.

18. Gottlieb JA, Baker LH, O'Bryan RM, et al.: Adriamycin used alone and in combination for soft tissue and bony sarcomas. Cancer Chemother Rep 6:271–282, 1975.

19. Klopp CT, Alford TC, Bateman J, et al.: Fractionated intraarterial cancer chemotherapy with methyl-bis-amine hydrochloride: a preliminary report. Ann Surg 132:811–832, 1950.

20. Ryan RF, Krementz ET Creech O, Winblad JN, Chamblee W, Creek H: Selected perfusion of isolated viscera with chemotherapeutic agents using an extracorporeal circuit. Surg Forum 8:158–161, 1957.

21. Stehlin JS, de Poli PD, Giovanella BC, Guiterrez AE, Anderson RF: Soft tissue sarcomas of the extremity: multidisciplinary therapy employing hyperthermic perfusion. Am J Surg 130:643–646, 1975.

22. McBride CM: Sarcoma of the limb: results of adjuvant chemotherapy using isolated limb perfusion. Arch Surg 109:304–308, 1974.

23. Stehlin JS: Hyperthermic perfusion with chemotherapy for cancers of the extremities. Surg Gynecol Obstet 129:305–308, 1969.

24. Haskell CM, Silverstein M, Rangel D, et al.: Multimodality cancer therapy in man: a pilot study of adriamycin by arterial infusion. Cancer 33:1485–1490, 1974.

25. Greco FA, Brereton HD, Kent H, Zimbler H, Merkly J, Johnson RE: Adriamycin and enhanced radiation reaction in normal esophagus and skin. Ann Intern Med 85:294–298, 1976.

26. Eilber FR, Townsend CM, Weisenberger TH, et al.: A clinicopathologic study: preoperative intraarterial adriamycin and radiation therapy for extremity soft tissue sarcomas. In: Management of primary soft tissue tumors: proceedings of the annual clinical conference on cancer, M.D. Anderson Hospital. Chicago: Year Book Medical, 1977, pp 411–422.

27. Morton DL, Eilber FR, Townsend CM, Grant TT, Mirra J, Weisenburger TH: Limb salvage from a multidisciplinary treatment approach for skeletal and soft tissue sarcomas of the extremity. Ann Surg 184:268–278, 1976.
28. Karakousis CP, Lopez R, Catane R, Rao U, Moore R, Holyoke ED: Intraarterial Adriamycin in the therapy of soft tissue sarcomas. J Surg Oncol 13:21–27, 1980.
29. Karakousis CP, Kanter DM, Park HC, et al.: Tourniquet infusion vs. hyperthermic infusion. Cancer 49:850–858, 1982.
30. Azzarelli A, Quagliuolo V, Audisio A, Bonfanta G, Andreola S, Gennari L: Intra-arterial Adriamycin followed by surgery for limb sarcomas: preliminary report. Eur J Cancer Clin Oncol 19:885–890, 1983.
31. DiPietro S, DePalo GM, Molinari R, Gennari L: Clinical trials with Adriamycin by prolonged arterial infusion. Tumori 56:233–244, 1970.
32. Anderson JH, Gianturco C, Wallace S: Experimental transcatheter intra-arterial infusion, occlusion chemotherapy. Invest Radiol 16:496–500, 1981.
33. Eilber FR, Morton DL, Eckardt JJ, Grant T, Weisenburger T: Limb salvage for skeletal and soft tissue sarcomas. Cancer 53:2579–2584, 1984.

9. Thermochemotherapy for soft tissue sarcoma

F. Di Filippo, G.L. Buttini, A.M. Calabro, S. Carlini, D. Gianarelli,
F. Moscarelli, F. Graziano, A. Cavallari, F. Cavaliere, and R. Cavaliere

During the last century, there have been many reports concerning the clinical application of hyperthermia in the treatment of human cancers [1–4]. The positive responses observed, although unpredictable and often evanescent, stimulated investigators to understand the action mechanism of heat better in order to apply hyperthermia rationally in the clinical setting. Not until the 1960s did in vitro and in vivo experiments demonstrate the selective heat sensitivity of cancer cells, and the first clinical applications of hyperthermic perfusion confirmed the effectiveness of heat in treating cancer [5].

After this first clinical experience, locoregional and whole body hyperthermic treatments largely expanded in clinical oncology and, more recently, new techniques such as nonionizing energies (microwave, radiofrequency, and ultrasound) have been employed in locoregional heating [6]. Notwithstanding advanced technology, two major limitations have been shown to hamper the therapeutic efficacy of hyperthermia: (a) difficulty in achieving a homogeneous cytotoxic temperature, simultaneously sparing normal tissues, and (b) thermoresistance [6–11]. These limitations prompted the combination of hyperthermia with other conventional therapies such as chemotherapy and radiotherapy in order to improve therapeutic efficacy [8–16]. As a matter of fact, many experimental in vitro and in vivo studies have shown that the association of heat with radiotherapy or chemotherapy results in a synergistic effect and, at present, only the combined treatments are clinically employed [7, 17–24].

Thermochemotherapy has been used in the treatment of a large variety of human cancers, and soft tissue sarcomas have been included in clinical trials.

In our personal experience, hyperthermia has been combined with chemotherapy in the treatment of locally aggressive or recurrent soft tissue sarcomas most frequently by perfusion in the case of limb localization, even if recently nonionizing energies have also been employed by many authors [23–25], with the same aim of improving regional control in association with conservative surgery and achieving palliation of unresectable tumors [17, 19, 21, 22, 26].

The potential benefit from systemic hyperthermia has also been studied in metastatic soft tissue sarcomas in order to evaluate the potentiation of the anticancer effect of the same drugs [18, 27–29]. This chapter reviews the clinical experience in treating primary and metastatic soft tissue sarcomas with hyperthermia associated with chemotherapy.

Pinedo, H.M., Verweij, J., eds. TREATMENT OF SOFT TISSUE SARCOMAS.
© Kluwer Academic Publishers, Boston. ISBN: 0-89838-391-9. All rights reserved.

Hyperthermia–chemotherapy interaction

It is a well-known fact that the association of hyperthermia and drugs can have an additive or synergistic effect [12–15, 30, 31]. Hyperthermia itself has a direct toxic effect on many cellular components or functions (DNA, RNA, protein synthesis, respiration) and can modify the membrane permeability or membrane transport, thus increasing drug uptake [12–14]. Furthermore, mild hyperthermia of 41°–42°C modifies tumor microcirculation, causing vasodilatation and increasing blood flow, resulting in a greater drug delivery to the tumor [32–34].

On the other hand, some antineoplastic drugs enhance the efficacy of heat in cancer killing by increasing the intracellular heat shock proteins that correlate with the appearance and decay of thermotolerance [35, 36]. 5-Thio-D-glucose and lonidamine, inhibitors of glucose metabolism, increase hyperthermia-induced cytotoxicity [37–39]; also quercetin-inhibiting lactate transport improves the tumoricidal effect of heat probably by exacerbating tumor cell acidosis [40–42].

Although our knowledge about the interaction of heat and chemotherapy is limited, many in vitro and in vivo experiments have provided useful information for the clinical application of thermochemotherapy. Hahn classified drugs into four categories by their interaction with heat [43–49]:

Classes	*Agent*
1. Drugs showing no threshold effect	Thiotepa, nitrosoureas, mitomycin, cisplatin
2. Drugs showing marked threshold effects	Doxorubicin, bleomycin, actinomycin
3. Thermosensitizers	Cysteamine, amphotericin B, AET, lidocaine, poliamine
4. Drugs showing no interaction with heat	Antimetabolites, methotrexate, 5-fluorouracil, vincristine, and vinblastine

To the first category belong cytotoxic agents that show a linear increase in cytotoxicity with increasing temperature [15, 40–44, 50]. The second category is represented by drugs that do not exhibit a linear cytotoxicity with heat, but do show a threshold temperature effect (42°–43°C) [12, 13, 46]. The third category of heat-interactive drugs consists of cytotoxic agents that have no cytotoxicity at 37°C, but become tumoricidal at higher temperatures [46–48]. Finally, there is a fourth group of drugs that show no change in cytotoxicity in a range of 37°–45°C [41, 46, 49].

The interactive mechanisms of hyperthermia–chemotherapy are quite complex and the association of the two modalities can result in a synergistic effect only if appropriately combined. Many in vitro and in vivo experiments have demonstrated that parameters most influencing the synergism are level of hyperthermia, sequence, and timing. Some drugs (cisplatin [CDDP] and L-phenylalinine mustard [LPAM]) show a synergistic effect only at a temperature of 42°C [16] as well as only with the simultaneous application of heat, other timing sequences producing only an additive or adverse effect [15, 16]. These experimental results have been confirmed in our clinical experience by hyperthermic antiblastic perfusion, the maximum complete response being observed only in the case of application of a temperature $\geq 41.5°C$ and a drug dose greater than or equal to the standard dose.

Techniques

Several techniques have been developed for local, regional, and whole body hyperthermia.

Locoregional heating has been clinically carried out with hyperthermic perfusion, ultrasound, and electromagnetic waves. The technique of hyperthermic perfusion has previously been described extensively [51]: basically, the blood circulating in an extracorporeal circuit equipped with oxygenator, pump, and heat exchanger acts as heat transfer in the region of the body where the tumor is located. More recently, new devices have been developed in clinical settings able to produce hyperthermia using different sources: (a) ultrasound operating in the frequency range of 0.3–6 MHz and (b) electromagnetic waves (microwave or radiofrequency) in the frequency range of 13–2450 MHz. Devices employing alternating electromagnetic fields can produce heat either by induction of electrical currents (inductive system) or by direct coupling of electromagnetic currents between applicators encompassing the tissues to be heated (capacitive system). Clinical application has demonstrated that many of these devices are quite effective for heating superficial lesions; but, on the contrary, none of the devices developed for deep heating have proved to be reliable so far [52, 53].

Whole body hyperthermia induction techniques have been extensively reviewed by Milligan [54]. Three techniques for delivery systemic hyperthermia are currently employed. The first utilizes direct contact between skin and some heat-transporting vehicles such as water, wax, or air. The second uses irradiation of body surface with nonionizing energy. The third technique is extracorporeal perfusion, which seems to be the most effective heating method for it allows a temperature of 41.5°–41.8°C to be reached within 30–90 min [53–59].

Local hyperthermia by perfusion

Regina elena institute experience. A total of 90 patients had been treated for soft tissue sarcomas of the extremities by July 1987. Table 1 shows the patient characteristics. At the time of referral, 55 (61.1%) of 90 patients had a recurrence of previously treated sarcomas. Most of the patients had developed

Table 1. Clinical characteristics of patients

Parameters	HP	HAP	Total (%)
Sex			
Male	13	38	51
Female	9	30	39
Age			
Median	41	52	52
(min-max)	8-72	14-76	8-76
Site			
Upper limb	9	15	24 (27%)
Arm	8	7	
Forearm	—	7	
Hand	1	1	
Lower Limb	13	53	66 (73%)
Thigh	8	30	
Leg	3	19	
Foot	2	4	
Histologic type			
Chondrosarcoma	4	1	5
Liposarcoma	6	23	29
m. f. histiocytoma	3	9	12
Fibrosarcoma	7	9	16
Sinovial sarcoma	—	7	7
Malignant schwannoma	—	4	4
Undetermined type	4	2	6
Rhabdomyosarcoma	—	3	3
Hemangiopericytoma	—	3	3
Dermatofibrosarcoma	—	2	2
Leiomyosarcoma	—	1	1
Angiosarcoma	1	1	2
Epithelial sarcoma	—	1	1

HP, hyperthermic perfusion; and HAP, hyperthermic antiblastic perfusion.

multiple recurrences, up to five in several cases, following surgery alone or multimodality treatments, as shown in Table 2.

Our first pilot study concerned 22 patients treated with hyperthermia as a single modality during limb perfusion. A minimum temperature of 42°C was always reached in all the tumoral areas and maintained for at least 2-4 h. Four postoperative toxic deaths occurred in this group. All of the remaining patients had a satisfactory tumor regression, enabling us to perform a delayed excision in 11 patients, whereas amputation was necessary in six patients. One patient refused further treatment and was soon lost to follow-up. The unacceptable mortality rate prompted us to lower the temperature applied, adding antineoplastic drugs to the perfusional circuit because of the synergism between the two modalities when applied simultaneously.

Since 1971, all patients (68 of 90) were treated by hyperthermic antiblastic

Table 2. Distribution of patients with recurrent disease according to previous treatment

Previous treatment	HP	HAP	Total
Excision	10	24	34
Radiotherapy	1	—	1
Excision + radiotherapy	5	11	16
Excision + chemotherapy	—	2	2
Excision + radiotherapy + chemotherapy	—	2	2
Total	16	39	55

HP, hyperthermic perfusion (22 patients); and HAP, hyperthermic antiblastic perfusion (68 patients). Patients with recurrent disease = 55/90 (61.1%).

perfusion (HAP) at muscle and tumor temperatures of 41°–41.5°C, never exceeding 41.8°C to avoid major complications. Melphalan (LPAM) (0.8 mg/kg body weight) and actinomycin D (DACT, or dactinomycin) (0.015 mg/kg body weight) were employed as antineoplastic drugs in the first series of 50 patients whereas, in the last 18 of 68, cisplatin (CDDP) with different schedules and dosages (2.5–3.2–5 mg/kg body weight, respectively) was employed during HAP [60].

Eight of the 68 patients presented with visceral metastases besides local relapse; therefore, they were treated with palliative intent and not included in any treatment protocol. Two patients died in the postoperative period; all of the remaining 58 patients underwent further therapy according to different protocols as follows: (a) HAP + surgery, (b) HAP + i.a. doxorubicin (DX) + surgery, and (c) HAP + radiotherapy + surgery.

Intra-arterial (i.a.) DX continuous infusion was generally initiated within 10 days after HAP; three cycles, 10 mg/day for 10 days each, were administered at 10-day intervals, followed by delayed surgery. Radiotherapy was performed by using an external beam source within 4 weeks after HAP administration; all patients received a dosage varying from 45 to 65 Gy, depending upon local tolerance, and delayed surgery was carried out 3–4 weeks later. Table 3 shows the stratification of 58 patients according to the stage of disease and treatment. It must be emphasized that 42 (72.4%) of 58 patients were classified as having stage III or IVA disease (American Joint Commission for Cancer Staging and End Results Reporting classification) [61].

Major complications occurred principally in the first series of 22 patients treated with hyperthermic perfusion. In all the patients, there were local complications such as limb swelling and blistering, and sometimes massive limb edema requiring fasciotomy or amputation. Four toxic deaths (18.8%) occurred in this group due to myocardial infarction, massive hemorrhage secondary to iliac artery rupture, and two acute renal failures.

In the group of 68 patients treated with HAP, the mortality rate was reduced to an acceptable minimum: two toxic deaths occurred (2.9%), both before 1975, due to hemorrhage after iliac arterial rupture and myocardial infarction,

Table 3. Distribution of patients treated with HAP according to stage and treatment protocols (patients included, 58)

| Treatment (HAP +) | Stages | | | | |
	I	II	III	IVA	Total
Excision	3	3	7	4	17
Amputation	—	1	3	9	13
DX i.a. infusion + excision	3	2	7	5	17
Radiotherapy + excision	2	2	3	4	11
Total	8	8	20	22	58

DX, doxorubicin; and HAP, hyperthermic antiblastic perfusion.

respectively. Regarding morbidity, only two amputations were directly related to perfusion in the group treated with HAP plus surgery. One patient treated with HAP plus i.a. DX infusion and surgery developed arteritis with progressive arterial insufficiency that required amputation 14 months after perfusion; one patient treated with HAP plus radiotherapy and surgery developed postactinic necrosis of the femur that required amputation 30 months after perfusion. Four patients had venous thrombosis that promptly recovered with standard therapy. Chronic renal insufficiency and moderate, but irreversible, neuropathy occurred in two patients treated with high-dose CDDP (5.0 mg/kg body weight) during HAP; since both local and systemic toxicities seemed strictly CDDP-dose related, in our experience 3.2 mg/kg body weight resulted in a safe therapeutic dose for temperatures not exceeding $41°-41.5°C$.

Patients were evaluated in terms of local control, percentage of conservative treatments, and disease-free and overall survival. Actuarial survivals were calculated using the Berkson–Gage method [62]. Functional results regarding limb salvage protocols were also evaluated.

When all patients were evaluated regardless of the treatment protocol, the 5- and 10-year disease-free and overall survivals were 41.8%–36.9% and 60.7%–48.8%, respectively. Of the 22 patients treated with hyperthermic perfusion followed by surgery, only 16 can be evaluated, as mentioned before, and the 5- and 10-year survival rates were 43.7% and 31.2%.

Only 58 of the 68 patients were treated with HAP have been evaluated. As far as the survival rate is concerned, our results confirm that long-term cure is strictly related to the stage regardless treatment protocol (Table 4). On the other hand, the assessment of results according to treatment sequence shows significant differences and, since the groups are well balanced for stage of disease, these differences should be correlated with the various effectiveness of treatments.

Regarding the 5- and 10-year locoregional control, results of treatment are reported in Table 5. HAP and surgery produced unsatisfactory results, whereas DX infusion or radiotherapy administered between perfusion and

117

Table 4. Survival according to stage of disease

Stage	Disease-free			Overall		
	5 years (%)		10 years (%)	5 years (%)		10 years (%)
I	83.3		62.5	100		75.0
II	59.2		59.2	71.4		71.4
III	32.5	$p=0.05$	32.5	73.0	$p=0.05$	58.4
IVA	32.1		32.1	33.8		33.8
		$p=0.01$			$p=0.4$	

118

Table 5. Locoregional control according to treatment

Treatment	5 years (%)	10 years (%)
HAP + surgery	75.1	75.1
HAP + DX i.a. infusion + surgery	84.2	˙84.2
HAP + XRT + surgery	100	100*

DX, doxorubicin; HAP, hyperthermic antiblastic perfusion; and XRT, radiotherapy.
* Control estimated at 8 years.

Table 6. Percentage of conservative surgery according to treatment protocol

Protocol	Conservative surgery	Demolitive surgery
HAP	17/30 (56.7%)	13/30 (43.3%)
HAP + DX infusion	15/16 (93.7%) ·	1/16[a] (6.3%)
HAP + XRT	10/10[b] (100%)	—

DX, doxorubicin; HAP, hyperthermic antiblastic perfusion; and XRT, radiotherapy.
[a] One patient excluded because of amputation for progressive arteritis 14 months after HAP.
[b] Patient excluded because of amputation for postactinic necrosis 30 months after HAP.

surgery yielded better locoregional control; the increased effectiveness of these two protocols also permitted a higher percentage of conservative surgery, as shown in Table 6. On the other hand, limb function was not impaired by these multistep treatments.

Table 7 presents the 5- and 10-year disease-free and overall survival rates. It must be emphasized that, also in terms of survival, more aggressive locoregional treatments produced better results.

Other clinical investigations. The wide clinical experience with hyperthermic antiblastic perfusion for soft tissue sarcoma should lead to an assessment of the real efficacy of HAP. Unfortunately, from the data reported in Table 8, it is readily apparent that there are many differences related to patient characteristics and treatment protocols. Different classifications have been used, as staging system and patients were not always stratified according to the stage of disease. Temperatures used during perfusion were not homogenous, ranging from 38° to 41°C.

Lethi et al. [21] and Stehlin et al. [22], after HAP administration, employed radiotherapy (30 and 50 Gy, respectively) before surgery; also the tumor was not always removed after HAP [21] even though all of the authors agree that surgery has to be performed after perfusion because this permits conservative rather then demolitive surgery.

Despite the above-mentioned difficulties in comparing results obtained by HAP, some positive conclusions can be made. This technique alone or associated with radiotherapy permitted a high percentage of conservative surgery

Table 7. Survival according to type of treatment

| Treatment | Disease free | | Overall | |
	5 years (%)	10 years (%)	5 years (%)	10 years (%)
HAP + surgery	32.1	32.1	46.8	46.8
HAP + DX infusion + surgery	49.6	33.1	74.5	42.6
HAP + XRT + surgery	58.3	58.3*	70.1	70.1*
		$p = 0.005$		
			NS	
			NS	

DX, doxorubicin; HAP, hyperthermic antiblastic perfusion; NS, not significant; p, Lee Desu test; and XRT, radiotherapy.
* 8 years.

Table 8. Soft tissue sarcomas of the extremities treated with HAP (LPAM + DACT)

Ref.	Stage	No. of patients	Protocol			Local relapse (%)	Systemic relapse (%)	% 5 year survival	Median follow-up (months)
			T°C	XRT	Conservative surgery (%)				
McBride (1978)	T <5 cm	110	39	—	100	15	18	~80	>60
	T >5 cm							~40	
Stehlin et al. (1984) [22]		65	38.8–40	+(65)	94	—	23	~72.7	?
Lehti et al. (1986) [21]	AJC								
	I–II	32							
	III–IV	32	>40	+(29)	100	11	NE	67	>60
Krementz (1986)	?	56	<41	—	100	21	NE	65	>60
Hoekstra (1987)	McBride								
	I–II	8	38–40	—	94	7	35	69	>156
	III	6							
Kruge (1987)	AJC	16	?	+(36)	?	11	?	64	?
	I–II								
	III–IV								

(94%–100%); the effectiveness of HAP in locoregional control of the disease is further suggested by the low incidence or recurrence (7%—21%) even in cases where demolitive surgery was not carried out. Finally, the 5-year over-all 69%–75% survival rate is quite satisfactory in relation to the high-risk patients treated.

Local hyperthermia by nonionizing energies

Local hyperthermia by nonionizing energies has been extensively applied in the treatment of superficial and deep lesions primarily in association with radiotherapy. However, there are only a few reports concerning the thermo-chemotherapy of soft tissue sarcomas.

Jabboury et al. [23] treated 12 advanced soft tissue sarcoma patients for a total of 20 lesions, half of which recurred after definitive radiotherapy; 13 lesions were superficial and seven were deep seated. Hyperthermia was carried out with radiofrequency and/or ultrasound. Seven lesions were treated with hyperthermia alone, whereas chemotherapy (CDDP) was added to treatment of 13 lesions. A temperature range of 41.5°–50°C was reached in all of lesions during all of the treatments. An objective response was observed in 50% of the lesions (four complete and six partial remissions), with a median duration of 4½ months. Interestingly, objective responses were observed in lesions treated with a higher temperature (46.6°C) while lower average temperatures (43.5°C) were attained in lesions that remained stable.

Storm et al. [25], in their multicenter trial of magnetic induction hyperther-mia (radiofrequency) reported the results in 130 soft tissue sarcoma patients treated with heat combined with chemotherapy or radiotherapy. Objective response was obtained in 23% of the patients; unfortunately it is not specified which treatments (thermoradiotherapy or thermochemotherapy) are responsi-ble for which responses. Nevertheless, it is interesting to note that, in patients who had previously failed to respond, the same chemotherapy caused tumor regression when combined with hyperthermia.

Systemic thermochemotherapy

Systemic thermochemotherapy has been employed in the treatment of meta-static soft tissue sarcomas. Whole body hyperthermia has been achieved by either extracorporeal circulation or warm blankets. Applied temperatures ranged 40°–43°C and were mantained for 2–5 hs. Antineoplastic drugs com-bined with hyperthermia were CDDP, BCNU, VP-16 (etoposide), CTX (Cytoxan, or cyclophosphamide), and DX, usually administered as soon as the target temperature was reached. Thus far, 34 patients have been treated with systemic thermochemotherapy. Complete response was observed in three patients (8.8%) and a partial response was obtained in eight patients (23.5%). The observed responses lasted from 2 to 12 months, with Gerad et al. [28] reporting the largest percentage of long-term responders.

Table 9. Systemic Thermochemotherapy: soft tissue sarcomas

Ref.	No. of patients	Technique	Protocol		Response		Duration of response (months)
			HT	CH	CR	PR	
Parks et al. (1980) [58]	1	EC 41.5–42 × 5 h	Cx	CDDP	—	—	—
Herman et al. (1982) [41]	3	EC–WB 42–42.5 × 2.5–3 h	Cx	CDDP or BCNU	—	1	2
Barlogie et al. (1979) [55]	1	WB 41.9–42 × 4 h	Cx	VP-16	—	1	—
Pettigrew et al. (1977) [59]	2	WAX 40–41 × 2 h	Cx	—	—	—	—
Bull et al. (1986) [27]	16	EC–WB 41.8 × 2 h	Cx	BCNU	1	4	4
Gerad et al. (1984) [28]	11	WB 41.8–43 × 2 h	Cx	DX CTX	2	2	12.3

EC, extracorporeal circulation; and WB, warm blankets.

Discussion and conclusions

There is substantial in vitro, in vivo, and clinical evidence indicating that hyperthermia has significant anticancer activity, especially when combined with chemotherapy. This combination has been employed in the treatment of soft tissue sarcomas that often are aggressive with a subclinical locoregional spread before systemic dissemination [63, 64].

Theoretically, hyperthermic antiblastic perfusion (HAP) seems to be a technique tailored to the treatment of soft tissue sarcomas of the extremities for several reasons: (1) Perfusional treatment involves the entire tumor-bearing limb, with possible control of micrometastatic foci. (2) The technique permits achievement of a homogeneous elevated temperature that can have a tumoricidal effect. (3) Concentrations of antineoplastic drugs 6–10 times greater than those given systemically can be injected into the perfusional circuit with an increased tumor drug uptake [60]. (4) Elevated temperature and drugs potentiate each other's activity. (5) Finally, the tumor mass "shrinkage" after HAP can permit conservative rather than demolitive surgery.

In our experience, HAP did not produce satisfactory locoregional control; conversely to what occurred in osteogenic sarcomas, this could be explained by the characteristics of the patients included in our trial. As matter of fact, many patients had been previously treated with surgery, radiotherapy, and/or chemotherapy: the first two treatments can reduce the blood circulation and drug uptake, due to sclerosis, while tumors previously treated with chemotherapy can become less responsive to further treatments.

Moreover, 23 (76.6%) of 30 patients in this series were in stage III–IVA, with a high risk of relapse. The association of i.a. DX infusion or radiotherapy with HAP before tumor removal permitted better locoregional control and a greater percentage of conservative surgery (Tables 5 and 6) without impairing limb function. The same results have been reported by Lethi et al. [21] and Stehlin et al. [22]. It is conceivable to hypothesize that the potential efficacy in tumor control can be further improved by using more specific drugs for soft tissue sarcomas, other than LPAM and DACT, which really demonstrated poor activity when used as single agents in treating soft tissue sarcomas [65–67]. Therefore, significant therapeutic gain could be derived from the use of DX, which, besides ascertained synergism with heat, has a well-documented tumor specific activity [19–22, 68].

As far as survival is concerned, trials employing HAP have obtained quite satisfactory results, rates ranging 65%–75% at 5 years. There are two main considerations in evaluating these results: (a) In most of the reported series, half of the patients had recurrences and it is known that local relapse is followed by pulmonary metastases in 30%–60% of these patients [63, 64]. (b) None of the patients treated with HAP underwent systemic chemotherapy which, in some clinical randomized trials, has proven to increase both disease-free and overall survival [69].

A reliable assessment of results obtained by local hyperthermia with nonionizing energies and systemic hyperthermia both associated with chemotherapy is difficult because too few and nonhomogeneous groups of patients have been treated with these modalities so far.

Difficulty in reaching elevated and homogeneous temperatures and reliable monitoring of heating during treatment of deep-seated tumors are the two main limitations of the hyperthermic treatment with nonionizing energies. Reaching an elevated an temperature is crucial in determining tumor response; in the report by Jabboury et al., objective responses were observed in lesions treated with high temperatures (46.6°C) while stable lesions were achieved at low average temperatures (43.5°C). These data are consistent with those reported by Storm et al. [25], who obtained objective responses when combining hyperthermia with the same drugs that had already been ineffective when normothermally administered.

A few pilot studies have been made on the clinical application of systemic hyperthermia and chemotherapy. Two main limitations hamper the potential effectiveness of these two modalities when systemically applied: level of hyperthermia and drug dose. In fact, the temperature usually cannot exceed 42°C (Table 9), to avoid cardiovascular and cerebral complications; on the other hand, the relatively low temperatures applied cannot be compensated for by elevated drug dosages because their systemic administration could be fatal to the patients. Nevertheless, complete and partial responses (11 of 31) have been reported by Bull et al. [27], Gerad et al. [28], Herman et al. [29], and Barlogie et al. [40] in previously treated patients, even though the response was not long lasting. In terms of cost benefit, it is difficult to assess the effectiveness of systemic thermochemotherapy in the treatment of metastatic soft tissue sarcomas, but at present further controlled investigations are warranted in selected patients and at experienced centers.

In conclusion, thermochemotherapy plays a major role in treating soft tissue sarcomas by achieving locoregional control by perfusion; whole body hyperthermic perfusion as well as nonionizing energies associated with chemotherapy require more technological hardware, and phase III studies are warranted to better select patients who can really benefit from these combined treatment modalities.

References

1. Busch W: Uber den Einfluss welchen heftiger erysipeln zuweilen auf organisierte Neubildungen ausuben. Verhandlungen des Naturhistorischer. Vereins Preussicher Rheinlands Westphalen 23:28–30, 1866.
2. Coley WB: The treatment of malignant tumours by repeated inoculations of erysipelas with a report of original cases. Am J Med Sci 105:487–511, 1893.
3. Rohdenburg GL, et al.: The effect of combined radiation and heat on neoplasms. Arch Surg 2:1548–1554, 1906.
4. Warren SL: Preliminary study of the effect of artificial fever upon hopeless tumour cases. AJR 33:75–87, 1935.
5. Cavaliere R, et al.: Selective heat sensitivity of cancer cells: biochemical and clinical studies.

Cancer 20:1351–1381, 1967.

6. Hunt JW: Applications of microwave, ultrasounds and radiofrequencies heating in vivo. In: Dethlefsen LA, Dewey WC (eds) Proceedings of the third international symposium on cancer therapy by hyperthermia, drugs and radiation. Bethesda MD; 447–456, 1984.

7. Gerner EW: Thermotolerance. In: Hyperthermia in cancer therapy, FK Storm, Boston: GK Hall, 1983, pp 141–162.

8. Dewey WC: Interaction of heat with radiation and chemotherapy. Cancer Res [Suppl] 44: 4714, 1984.

9. Gillette EG: Clinical use of thermal enhancement and therapeutic gain for hyperthermia combined with radiation or drugs. Cancer Res [Suppl] 44:4836, 1984.

10. Field SB, et al.: Thermotolerance: a review of observations and possible mechanism. Natl Cancer Inst Monogr 61:193–201, 1982.

11. Nielsen OS, et al.: Arrhenius analysis of survival curves from thermotolerant and step-down heated L1A2 cells in vitro. Radiat Res 91:468–482, 1982.

12. Hahn GM: Hyperthermia and cancer. New York: Plenum, 1982, pp 74–85.

13. Hahn GM, et al.: Thermochemotherapy: synergism between hyperthermia (42–43) and adriamycin (or bleomycin) in mammalian cell inactivation. Proc Natl Acad Sci USA 72: 937–940, 1975.

14. Hahn GM: Potential for therapy of drugs and hyperthermia. Cancer Res 39:2264–2268, 1979.

15. Marmor JE: Interactions of hyperthermia and chemotherapy in animals. Cancer Res 39: 2269–2276, 1979.

16. Greco C, et al.: Effect of sequential application of hyperthermia and chemotherapy on the survival of a thermoresistant human melanoma cell line. Cancer Biochem Biophys 9:223–232, 1987.

17. Moricca G, et al.: Hyperthermic treatment of tumors: experimental and clinical applications. Recent Results Cancer Res 59:112–151, 1977.

18. Bull JMC: An update of the anticancer effects of a combination of chemotherapy and hyperthermia. Cancer Res [Suppl] 44:4853–4856, 1984.

19. Schraffordt Koops HS, et al.: Isolated regional perfusion in the treatment of soft tissue sarcomas of the extremities. Clin Oncol 2:245–252, 1976.

20. Karakousis CP, et al.: Touniquet infusion versus hyperthermic perfusion. Cancer 49:850–858, 1982.

21. Lehti PM, et al.: Improved survival for soft tissue sarcoma of the extremities by regional hyperthermic perfusion, local excision and radiation therapy. Surg Gynecol Obstet 162: 149–152, 1986.

22. Stehlin JS, et al.: 15 year's experience with hyperthermic perfusion for treatment of soft tissue sarcoma and malignant melanoma of the extremities. In: Vaeth JM (ed) Hyperthermia and radiation therapy/chemotherapy in the treatment of cancer. San Francisco, 1984, pp 177–182.

23. Jabboury K, et al.: Local hyperthermia for resistant soft tissue sarcoma [abstr]. In: 34th annual meeting of the Radiation Research Society, Las Vegas, April 1986, p 18.

24. Bicher HI, et al.: Clinical thermoradiotherapy. In: Storm FK (ed) Hyperthermia in cancer therapy. Boston: GK Hall, 1983.

25. Storm FK, et al.: Magnetic induction hyperthermia: results of a 5 year multiinstitutional national cooperative trial in advanced cancer patients. Cancer 55:2677–2687, 1985.

26. Di Filippo F, et al.: Role of hyperthermic perfusion as a first step in the treatment of soft tissue sarcoma of the extremities. World J Surg 12:332–339, 1988.

27. Bull JMC, et al.: An update of whole body hyperthermia + BCNU in advanced sarcoma [abstr]. Proc Am Soc Clin Oncol 5:144, 1986.

28. Gerad H, et al.: Doxorubicun, cyclophosphamide and W.B.H. for treatment of advanced soft tissue sarcomas. Cancer 53:2585–2591, 1984.

29. Herman TS, et al.: W.B.H. and chemotherapy for treatment of patients with advanced refractory malignancies. Cancer Treat Rep 66:259–265, 1982.

30. Har-Kedar I, et al.: Experimental and clinical aspects of hyperthermia applied to the treatment of cancer with special reference to the role of ultrasonic and microwave heating. Adv Radiat Biol 6:229–266, 1976.
31. Hahn GM: Interactions of drugs and hyperthermia in vitro and in vivo. In: Streffer C (ed) Proceedings of the second international symposium on cancer therapy by hyperthermia and radiation. Baltimore: Urban and Schwarzenberg, 1978, pp 72–79.
32. Song CW: Effect of local hyperthermia on blood flow and microenvironment: a review. Cancer Res [Suppl] 44:4721–4730, 1984.
33. Emami B, et al.: Histopathological study on the effects of hyperthermia on microvasculature. Int J Radiat Oncol Biol Phys 7:343–348, 1981.
34. Olch A, et al.: Blood flow in human tumors during hyperthermic therapy: demonstration of vasoregulation and an applicable physiological model. J Surg Oncol 23:125–132, 1983.
35. Li GC, et al.: Correlation between synthesis of heat shock proteins and development of thermotolerance in Chinese hamster fibroblasts. Proc Natl Acad Sci USA 79:3219–3222, 1982.
36. Tomasovic SP, et al.: Heat stress proteins and thermal resistance in rat mammary tumor cells. Radiat Res 70:610–611, 1977.
37. Reinhold HS, et al.: Enhancement of thermal damage to sandwich tumors by additional treatment. In: Arcangeli G, Mauro F (eds) Proceedings of the first meeting of the European Group on Hyperthermia in Radiation Oncology. Milan: Massom, 1980, pp 179–183.
38. Kim JH, et al.: Lonidamine: a hyperthermic sensitizer of HeLa cells in culture and of Meth-A tumor in vivo. Oncology [Suppl 1] 41:30–35, 1984.
39. Kim JH, et al.: Quercetin, an inhibitor of lactate transport and a hyperthermic sensitizer of HeLa cells. Cancer Res 44:102–106, 1984.
40. Barlogie B, et al.: In vitro thermochemotherapy of human colon cancer cells with CDDP and mitomycin C. Cancer Res 40:1165–1168, 1980.
41. Herman TS: Effect of temperature on the cytotoxicity of vindesine, amsacrine and mitoxantrone. Cancer Treat Rep 67:1019–1022, 1983.
42. Johnson HA, et al.: Thermal enhancement of thiotepa cytotoxicity. J Natl Cancer Inst 50: 903–908, 1973.
43. Joiner MC, et al.: Response of two mouse tumors to hyperthermia with CCNU or melphalan. Br J Cancer 45:19–26, 1982.
44. Lees DE, et al.: Internal organ hypoxia during hyperthermic cancer therapy in humans. In: Proceedings of the third international symposium on cancer therapy by hyperthermic drugs and radiation, Fort Collins CO, 1980, p 93.
45. Meyn RE, et al.: Thermal enhancement of DNA damage in mammalian cells treated with CDDP. Cancer Res 40:1136–1139, 1980.
46. Bleehan NM, et al.: Interaction of hyperthermia and the hypoxic cell sensitizer RO-07-0582 on the EMT6 mouse tumor. Br J Cancer 35:299–306, 1977.
47. Kapp DS, et al.: Thermosensitization by sulfhydryl compounds of exponentially growing Chinese hamster cells. Cancer Res 29:4630–4635, 1979.
48. Robins IH, et al.: Systemic lidocaine enhancement of hyperthermia-induced tumor regression in transplantable murine tumor models. Cancer Res 43:3187–3191, 1983.
49. Herman TS, et al.: Reversal of resistance to methotrexate by hyperthermia in Chinese hamster ovary cells. Cancer Res 41:3840–3843, 1981.
50. Mimnaugh EG, et al.: Effect of W.B.H. on the deposition and metabolism of ADR in rabbits. Cancer Res 38:1420–1425, 1978.
51. Cavaliere R, et al.: Regional perfusion hyperthermia. In: Storm FK (ed) Hyperthermia in cancer therapy. Boston: GK Hall, 1983.
52. Cheung AY, et al.: Deep local hyperthermia for cancer therapy: external electromagnetic and ultrasound techniques. Cancer Res [Suppl] 44:4736–4744, 1984.
53. Atkinson ER: Hyperthermia techniques and instrumentation. In: Storm FK (ed) Hyperthermia in cancer therapy. Boston: GK Hall, 1983, pp 233–255.

54. Milligan AJ: Whole body hyperthermia induction techniques. Cancer Res [Suppl] 44: 4869–4872, 1984.
55. Barlogie B, et al.: Total body hyperthermia with and without chemotherapy for advanced human neoplasms. Cancer Res 39:1481–1489, 1979.
56. Bull JM, et al.: Whole body hyperthermia: now a feasible addition to cancer treatment. Proc Am Assoc Cancer Res 19:405, 1978.
57. Larkin JM, et al.: Systemic thermotherapy: description of a method and physiologic tolerance in clinical subjects. Cancer 40:3155–3159, 1977.
58. Parks LC, et al.: Treatment of far advanced bronchogenic carcinoma by extracorporeally induced systemic hyperthermia. J Thorac Cardiovasc Surg 28:467–477, 1979.
59. Pettigrew RT, et al.: Whole body hyperthermia combined with chemotherapy in the treatment of advanced human cancer. In: Streffer C (ed) Cancer therapy by hyperthermia and radiation. Baltimore: Urban and Schwarzenberg, 1978, pp 326–327.
60. Di Filippo F, et al.: Isolated hyperthermic perfusion with CDDP in the treatment of limb tumors: phase I study—toxicity and pharmacokinetics. J Exp Clin Cancer Res 6:257–265, 1987.
61. Russel WO, et al.: A clinical and pathological staging system for soft tissue sarcomas. Cancer 40:1562–1570, 1977.
62. Berkson J, Gage RP: Calculation of survival rates for cancer. Mayo Clin Proc 25:270–286, 1950.
63. Cantin J, et al.: The problem of local recurrences after treatment of soft tissue sarcoma. Ann Surg 168:47–53, 1968.
64. Heise HW, et al.: Recurrence-free survival time for surgically treated soft tissue sarcoma patients: multivariate analysis of five prognostic factors. Cancer 57:172–177, 1986.
65. Cruz AB, et al.: Combination chemotherapy for soft tissue sarcomas: a phase II study. J Surg Oncol 11:313–323, 1979.
66. Greenall MS, et al.: Chemotherapy for soft tissue sarcoma. Surg Gynecol Obstet 162: 193–198, 1986.
67. Verweij J, Pinedo HM: Chemotherapy in advanced soft tissue sarcoma In: Pinedo HM, Verweij J (eds) Clinical management of soft tissue sarcoma. Boston: Martinus Nijhoff, 1986, pp 81–88.
68. Eilber FR, et al.: Limb salvage for skeletal and soft tissue sarcomas: multidisciplinary preoperative therapy. Cancer 53:2579–2584, 1984.
69. Rosenberg SA, et al.: Sarcomas of the soft tissue and bone. In: Devita, Hellman, Rosenberg (eds) Cancer: principles and practice of oncology. Philadelphia: JB Lippincott, 1982, pp 1036–1093.

Index